ACE Inhibitors in Hypertension
A Guide for General Practitioners

ACE Inhibitors in Hypertension
A Guide for General Practitioners

Dr Gillian Strube
Medical Advisor to West Sussex FHSA
and
Dr George Strube
Medical Audit Facilitator, West Sussex FHSA

KLUWER ACADEMIC PUBLISHERS
DORDRECHT / BOSTON / LONDON

Distributors

---

for the United States and Canada: Kluwer Academic Publishers, PO Box 358,
Accord Station, Hingham, MA 02018-0358, USA
for all other countries: Kluwer Academic Publishers Group, Distribution
Center, PO Box 322, 3300 AH Dordrecht, The Netherlands

British Library Cataloguing in Publication Data

Strube, Gillian
   ACE inhibitors in hypertension: a guide for general practitioners.
   1. Humans. Circulatory system. Drug therapy
   I. Title II. Strube, George
   616.1061

   ISBN 0-7923-8963-8

Published in the United Kingdom by Kluwer Academic Publishers,
PO Box 55, Lancaster, UK.

Kluwer Academic Publishers BV incorporates the publishing programmes of
D. Reidel, Martinus Nijhoff, Dr W. Junk and MTP Press.

Printed in Great Britain by Billings and Sons, Worcester.

Contents

1	Introduction	1
2	Physiology	3
3	Cardiac and vascular implications of hypertension: the need for treatment	17
4	Diagnosis and assessment of essential hypertension	31
5	The management of patients with hypertension	43
6	The ACE inhibitor drugs: history and pharmacology	55
7	Safety and side-effects of ACE inhibitors	69
8	Special patient groups	75
9	Combination therapy with ACE inhibitors	97
10	Conclusion	99
	Further reading	101
	Index	103

1

Introduction

ACE inhibitors are one of the most exciting and interesting of recent medical developments. They fit the patho-physiological processes of cardiovascular disease with fascinating precision and are a constant stimulus to the acquisition of greater understanding of the mechanisms involved and of the mode of action of the drugs themselves. There is still much to be learned, especially about the wider effects of the drugs, their precise mode and site of action and about differences between the different preparations. ACE inhibitors are of proven benefit to patients with chronic congestive heart failure and are the latest in the series of drugs used in the treatment of hypertension.

Interest in the treatment of hypertension has paralleled the development of hypotensive drugs and the realisation that long-term prognosis could be significantly improved. The treatment of hypertension has progressed in stages following the development of a succession of increasingly effective drugs, each allowing a greater proportion of patients to be treated with fewer and fewer side-effects.

First, the ganglion-blocking agents such as hexamethonium and guan-ethidine transformed the outlook for patients with malignant hypertension but proved too unpleasant for routine use in other forms of hypertension. Next came the rauwolfia group and methyldopa which extended the range of patients treated and reduced the incidence of stroke in hypertensives. The major breakthrough in routine long-term treatment of moderate hyper-tension came with the development of designer drugs and the introduction of β-blockers. These, used alone and in combination with thiazide diuretics and with calcium antagonists, still form the basis of the standard treatment in uncomplicated patients.

However it is by no means a perfect regime. Many people, such as those suffering from asthma or heart failure, cannot take β-blockers. Some suffer side-effects. Others, such as diabetics and the elderly, do not benefit overall because of unwelcome secondary effects.

It is likely that ACE inhibitors will solve the problem of treating hypertension in most of these patients and therefore have a major role to play in modern therapy.

In addition, although the incidence of stroke associated with hypertension has continued to fall, that of myocardial infarction has remained unchanged. If ACE inhibitors were found to solve this problem, then they might become the drugs of first choice in the treatment of the majority of hypertensive patients.

In this book we remind readers of the renin–angiotensin–aldosterone system, the pathophysiology of hypertension and of where ACE inhibitors fit into the general picture.

2

Physiology

Physiological control of blood pressure

If the process and effects of disease are to be understood and remedies appropriately applied, it is necessary to bear in mind the normal physiology.

Systemic blood pressure is a product of left ventricular output (LVO) and systemic vascular resistance (SVR), also called peripheral resistance.

$$LVO \times SVR = BP$$

This is Ohm's law which states that

$$Flow\ (LVO) = \frac{pressure\ (BP)}{resistance\ (SVR)}$$

The SVR is dependent on the diameter of the arterioles. In health, this depends solely on the tone of smooth muscle in the arterioles which is controlled by the homeostatic mechanisms described below.

If the SVR rises, the blood pressure rises, as long as the left ventricle can keep the output the same. The blood pressure also rises if the cardiac output increases but the peripheral resistance stays the same.

There are often changes in both parameters. For instance, during exercise, the peripheral resistance falls due to arteriolar dilatation and increased blood flow to skeletal muscles but the cardiac output rises so much that the blood pressure rises. This is such a consistent response that it can be used as a measure of left ventricular function. If, during an exercise test, the blood pressure fails to rise, this is taken as evidence of poor left ventricular function and is a poor prognostic sign.

The status quo is maintained by a complex system of inter-related feedback mechanisms known as homeostatic mechanisms.

These include the autonomic nervous system (with its two components, the sympathetic and parasympathetic systems) and the renin–angiotensin system. Both of these involve circulating and local, tissue-based humoral agents.

The autonomic nervous system

The behaviour of the cardiovascular system is regulated, to a great extent, by the competing or balancing effects of the sympathetic and parasympathetic divisions of the autonomic nervous system.

The sympathetic nervous system

Sympathetic activity is increased by exercise, by stress and by a fall in systemic blood pressure, detected by baroreceptors in the carotid sinus and aortic arch and transmitted by the nerves of the sympathetic nervous system.

These effects are mediated by catecholamines, such as noradrenaline, which are produced at sympathetic nerve endings and in the adrenal medulla.

The production of catecholamines by the adrenal medulla is also increased by high levels of angiotensin II (p. 10).

The effects of increased sympathetic tone are complex. They can be divided into α and β adrenergic effects, some of which are shown in Table 2.1.

Table 2.1 Some α and β adrenergic effects

	α effects	β effects
	Vasoconstriction	Vasodilatation
	Intestinal muscle relaxation	Heart: increased force and rate; arrhythmias
	Pupillary dilatation	Bronchial relaxation
Noradrenaline	+++	+
Adrenaline	+	+++

The α and β effects can be further subdivided into α_1, α_2, β_1 and β_2 effects (Figures 2.1 and 2.2).

4

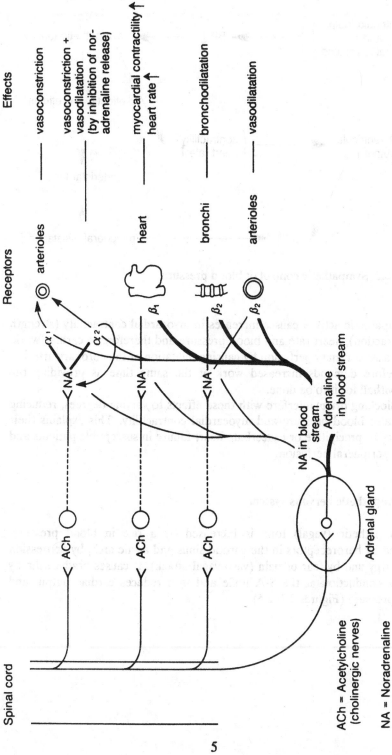

Figure 2.1 α and β effects of sympathetic nervous system

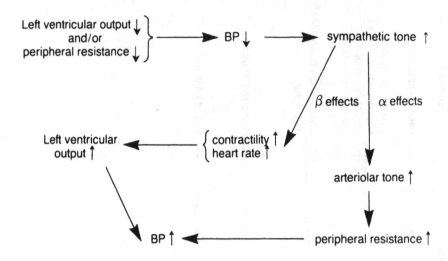

Figure 2.2 Sympathetic control of blood pressure

Sympathetic activity causes increases in myocardial contractility (strength of contraction), heart rate and blood pressure and therefore in cardiac work. It increases coronary perfusion by causing dilatation of the coronary arteries. It therefore demands increased work at the same time as providing the wherewithall for it to be done.

β-Blocking drugs interfere with these effects to varying degrees, reducing heart rate, blood pressure and myocardial contractility. This explains their tendency to precipitate or exacerbate heart failure in susceptible patients and reduce peripheral perfusion.

Parasympathetic nervous system

Parasympathetic (vagal) tone is increased by a rise in blood pressure, detected by baroreceptors in the carotid sinus and aortic arch, by depression or lethargy and by fear or pain (vaso-vagal attack). It causes bradycardia by slowing conduction at the S-A node and thus reduces cardiac output and blood pressure (Figures 2.3–2.5).

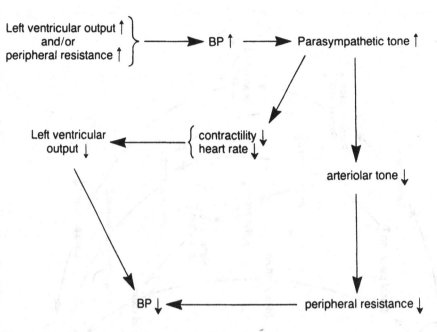

Figure 2.3 Parasympathetic control of blood pressure

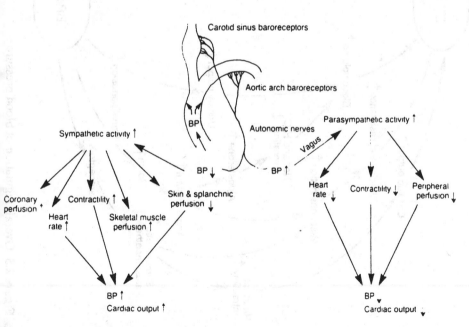

Figure 2.4 The autonomic nervous system

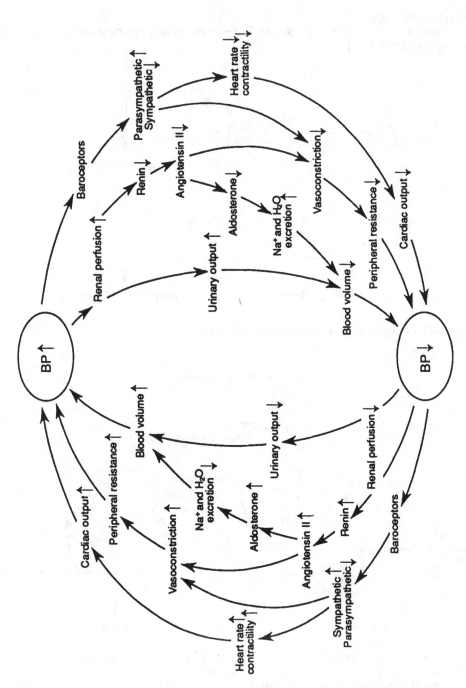

Figure 2.5 Overall regulation of blood pressure

The renin–angiotensin–aldosterone system (RAAS)

Angiotensinogen is secreted by the liver and is taken up by all tissues.

Renin is released into the circulation in response to low blood pressure and low serum sodium, detected by juxtaglomerular cells in the kidney and by activation of the sympathetic nervous system.

Angiotensinogen forms angiotensin I in the presence of renin and this is further changed into the active hormone angiotensin II in the presence of angiotensin converting enzyme (ACE).

The rate of production of angiotensin II is related to the level of angiotensinogen. This is increased by oestrogens, steroids and thyroid hormones, which may be linked to the observation that oral contraceptive and systemic steroid administration cause hypertension in some people.

This systemic endocrine mechanism appears to be supplemented by a local RAA system within blood vessels of peripheral tissues.

When this acts within the cells which produce it, it is said to have an autocrine effect and when it acts in neighbouring cells, the effect is said to be paracrine.

This series of events takes place in all tissues but is of greatest significance in the kidney, where it regulates glomerular filtration rate (GFR) by its effects on blood flow in the nephron. It also controls blood volume by its effects on tubular resorption, through the action of aldosterone (see below).

Glomerular filtration rate depends on the pressure in the capillaries of Bowman's capsule. This in turn depends on the systemic blood pressure and relative pressures in the afferent and efferent arterioles (see Figure 2.6). Angiotensin II causes constriction of the efferent arteriole, increasing the pressure in the capillaries of Bowman's capsule and therefore the GFR.

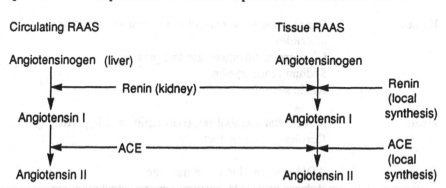

Figure 2.6 Inter-relationship between circulating and tissue renin–angiotensin–aldosterone systems.

It is a powerful vasoconstrictor and has a direct effect on peripheral arteriolar tone. This increases peripheral resistance and the blood pressure rises. The local, tissue-based RAA system appears to be more important in this than the endocrine (circulating) system. This might explain the observation that ACE inhibitors have as great a hypotensive effect in patients with normal or low serum renin levels as in those with high renin levels.

Thus the RAA system safeguards GFR in the face of reduced renal arterial pressure in two ways: by increasing systemic blood pressure and by the local effect on capillary circulation in Bowman's capsule.

ACE inhibitors interrupt this sequence of events by preventing the formation of angiotensin II.

Patients with renal artery stenosis depend on the RAA system to maintain renal function and this may be jeopardised by the administration of ACE inhibitors.

Angiotensin II has diverse effects on many tissues (Table 2.2). It increases the rate and strength of contraction of the heart. Angiotensin II also causes the release of catecholamines from the renal medulla, of aldosterone from the adrenal cortex and of antidiuretic hormone (ADH) from the posterior pituitary.

Table 2.2 Actions of angiotensin II

Tissue	Effect
Vasculature	Vasoconstriction Vascular hypertrophy
Kidney	Renal blood flow: control of afferent and efferent arterioles Glomerular filtration rate and pressure Sodium reabsorption Renin secretion
Heart	Myocardial metabolism, contractility and hypertrophy Coronary vascular tone
Brain	ADH release: thirst: salt appetite Release of ACTH, vasopressin and catecholamines
Adrenals	Catecholamine release (medulla) Aldosterone release

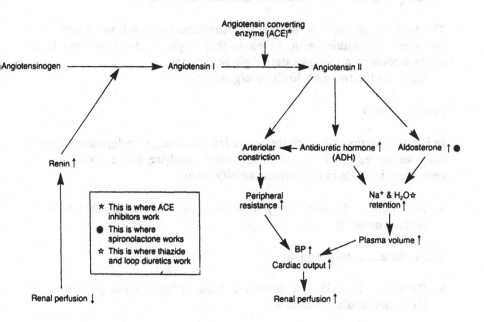

Figure 2.7 The renin–angiotensin–aldosterone system

Aldosterone and ADH both cause sodium and water retention and therefore increase plasma volume by their action on the renal tubules. ADH increases thirst and appetite for salt. Aldosterone also causes potassium loss.

Activation of this system therefore leads to increased blood pressure, plasma volume and renal perfusion. This in turn leads to a reduction in renin levels as the stimulus to its release is removed.

The kallikrein–kinin system

Bradykinin stimulates the synthesis and release of vasodilator prostaglandins and is itself a vasodilator hormone.

Angiotensin converting enzyme (ACE) is identical to the enzyme, kininase II, which is involved in the breakdown of bradykinin.

The activity of ACE therefore promotes vasoconstriction through two mechanisms, the RAA and the kallikrein–kinin systems.

The conflict of survival mechanisms and disease processes

The basic homeostatic or feedback mechanisms work well when applied to the needs of primitive man, in whom they originally developed and in his modern counterpart facing external physical threat.

Consider the two most likely emergencies:

Intense exertion

In intense exertion, which might be needed in hunting or in fighting or fleeing from an aggressor, dilatation of arterioles supplying active tissues and an immediate increase in sympathetic activity ensure:

1. Distribution of blood supply to where it is most needed (brain, heart, skeletal muscle);

2. Increase in cardiac output;

3. Reduction in fluid loss (resulting from reduced renal perfusion and increased tubular resorption).

Haemorrhage

After haemorrhage, the sympathetic system is stimulated by the fall in blood pressure. The reduction in cardiac output and renal perfusion triggers the renin–angiotensin system. This has a dual role:

1. IMMEDIATELY, the vasopressor effect of angiotensin II helps to keep the blood pressure up in the short term;

2. LATER, the increase in plasma volume allows the circulation to be maintained while long-term reparative work takes place.

GFR is safeguarded by the RAAS described above.

All this involves a massive increase in cardiac work and increase in peripheral resistance, increasing blood pressure. It depends on a healthy myocardium as well as on structurally normal valves and vasculature and on the effect of feedback in reversing the mechanism when it is no longer of benefit.

In disease, these mechanisms may work to the detriment of the individual.

The body reacts to every fall in blood pressure as if it were due to haemorrhage, as when it demands increased work from the heart following myocardial infarction.

Whilst the precise role of the homeostatic mechanisms in causing

12

hypertension is not clear, it does appear that interfering with them lowers blood pressure.

It is for this reason that some of the most effective drugs used in treating hypertension are those which block homeostatic mechanisms. They include β-blockers, anti-aldosterone agents, α-blockers, calcium-channel blockers and angiotensin-converting enzyme (ACE) inhibitors (Figure 2.8).

Blood fats

Cholesterol and triglycerides are the most important fats, or lipids, in the blood.

Cholesterol

Cholesterol is used in the body for the synthesis of cell membranes, hormones and bile acids. It forms a part of our diet and is also synthesised in all tissues but mainly in the liver. It is insoluble in water and is transported combined with protein in the form of various lipoprotein fractions.

Total cholesterol (TC) is the most common measurement of cholesterol in the blood and should ideally be less than 5.2 mmol/L; the lipoprotein fractions (Table 2.3) can be separated according to their density:

1. Low-density lipoproteins (LDL) supply cholesterol to the peripheral tissues. If present in excess, they are deposited in the arterial walls and contribute to the formation of atheroma. Thus, a high level of LDL in the serum is associated with a high risk of ischaemic heart disease. Ideal levels are less than 4.0 mmol/L.

2. High-density lipoproteins (HDL) contain esterified cholesterol, which has been removed from the peripheral tissues and is on the way back to the liver to be excreted in the bile. A high concentration of HDL is associated with a low risk of ischaemic heart disease. Ideal levels are higher than 1.15 mmol/L.

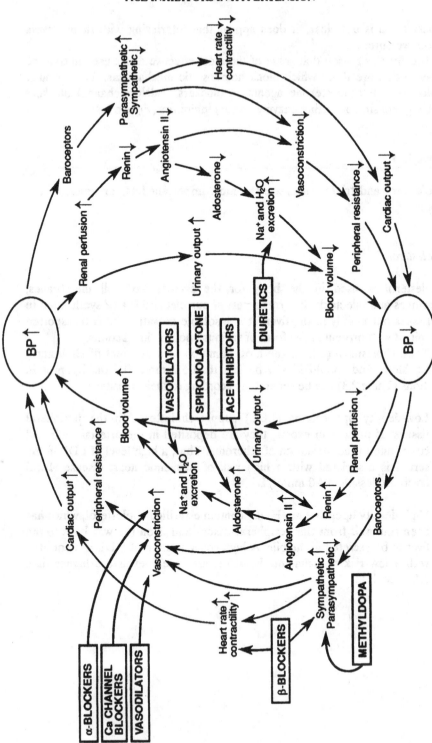

Figure 2.8 Effects of drugs on the physiological control of blood pressure

Table 2.3 Types of lipoprotein

Lipoprotein	Characteristics
LDL	Rich in cholesterol High level associated with high risk of IHD Lowering level can reduce risk of IHD
HDL	Contains esterified cholesterol [safe] High level associated with low risk of IHD
VLDL	Rich in triglycerides

Triglycerides

Triglycerides are also derived from dietary fat but they can be synthesised in the liver from carbohydrates and free fatty acids. These are transported to peripheral tissues by very-low-density lipoproteins (VLDL) in response to high carbohydrate and alcohol intake. They are not directly related to high risk of coronary artery disease but have an adverse influence on blood clotting factors. Triglycerides are broken down in muscle and adipose tissue to glycerol and free fatty acids, which are used for energy and storage. Dietary triglycerides are carried in chylomicrons, which give the serum a turbid appearance after a fatty meal.

The relationship between total cholesterol and HDL/LDL cholesterol is expressed in the Friedwald formula which also takes into account the level of triglyceride (but ignores the very small contribution made by VLDL cholesterol):

$$LDLC = TC - HDLC - \frac{triglycerides}{2.2} \quad (mmol/L)$$

When calculating the cardiovascular risk, the total cholesterol/HDL cholesterol ratio is sometimes used:

$$Ratio = TC/HDLC$$

The normal range is 3 to 6. Higher figures carry an increased risk.

3

Cardiac and vascular implications of hypertension: the need for treatment

Pathophysiology

The two main homeostatic mechanisms described in Chapter 2 have the effect of maintaining the blood pressure under physiological conditions.

1. The sympathetic nervous system acts in response to:

- a reduction in blood pressure detected by the baroreceptors in the aortic arch and carotid bodies;

- stress (e.g. pain or fear): the fight/flight mechanism;

- exercise.

The rise in blood pressure in these circumstances results from a selective increase in peripheral arteriolar constriction and also an increase in contractility of the myocardium.

2. The renin–angiotensin–aldosterone (RAA) system is stimulated by reduced renal blood flow. Angiotensin II is a powerful vasopressor, causing peripheral vasoconstriction. It also causes increased secretion of aldosterone resulting in sodium and fluid retention.

The effects of these mechanisms are normally short term, lasting only a matter of hours or days.

In patients with hypertension, the actions appear to persist.

Persistent activation of these systems results in hyperplasia and proliferation of smooth muscle cells in the walls of small arteries, increasing peripheral resistance and therefore blood pressure.

These changes in the vessel walls are mediated by the increase in intravascular pressure, the neuro-humoral mechanisms of the sympathetic and RAA systems outlined above and possibly also by other hormones, including insulin and growth factor.

The thickened small arteries in turn seem to show hyper-reactivity to the vasopressor stimuli of the sympathetic and RAA systems so that a self-perpetuating situation is generated.

Causative factors in hypertension

There are a number of factors which are known to be important in the prognosis of patients with hypertension. Some of them are also involved in the aetiology of hypertension but the relationships are complex and not well understood.

They include all the risk factors for ischaemic heart disease:

> Smoking
> Alcohol consumption
> Diabetes
> Hyperlipidaemia
> Family history
> Male sex
> Obesity
> Stress
> Atheroma
> Left ventricular hypertrophy
> Salt intake
> Oral contraceptive use

Most of these factors influence each other or have complex causal inter-relationships (Figure 3.1).

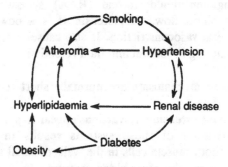

Figure 3.1 Circular effects of mechanisms

The importance of these factors varies from one individual to another and their significance is easier to prove at population than at individual level.

This emphasises the importance of health education to reduce the risk of cardiovascular disease in the population as a whole (see Chapter 5).

Some of these factors are themselves amenable to treatment while others are unalterable. Thus, whilst nothing can be done about anyone's sex or family history, smoking, alcohol consumption, hyperlipidaemia and obesity can be treated and diabetic control can often be improved, if the patient is cooperative.

It may be that any treatment of hypertension is better than none in preventing stroke, but in certain groups the decision to use drugs and the choice of drug is of particular importance and may influence the risk of ischaemic heart disease.

The choice of drugs in people with additional risk factors is especially important. For instance, it is better to avoid thiazide diuretics in diabetics, and β-blockers tend to cause an increase in serum triglycerides and make it more difficult to improve the lipid profile overall.

Alcohol

Alcohol abuse is of aetiological importance in some people. Since it is impossible to know who they are, it is sensible to advise all hypertensives to drink moderately, if at all. Low alcohol consumption seems to make it easier to control hypertension.

Salt intake

The ability of the kidneys to excrete sodium is impaired in at least some people with hypertension and some hypertensives can reduce their blood pressure by reducing salt intake. It does not work for everyone but it is presumably an integral part of the cause of the hypertension in those for whom it does.

Renin levels

Some patients with hypertension have raised serum renin levels but others do not. However, ACE inhibitors work equally well in both groups. This may be because local, tissue RAA systems are active in hypertensive people who have normal or low circulating (endocrine) renin or alternatively the kallikrein–kinin system (p. 11) is of greater importance. Hypertension in these patients may therefore be independent of the endocrine RAA system.

Smoking

Hypertension affects non-smokers as well as smokers but it makes a significant difference to the prognosis as well as to the effectiveness of treatment. There is no evidence that mild hypertensives who continue to smoke benefit from drug treatment at all. Smoking has an adverse influence on blood fats.

It also influences the choice of medication: it may be better to start with a thiazide diuretic than a β-blocker in a smoker, if the standard regime is being followed (see Chapter 5).

Stress

Short-term stress has the effect of raising the blood pressure in normal people. It is part of the fight and flight mechanism. It has been postulated that, in people who are subject to frequent or continuous stress, the baroreceptors are reset at a higher level. This would have the effect of making their 'normal' blood pressure pathologically high and be a cause of their hypertension.

There is also evidence that stress causes an increase in the low-density lipoprotein fractions of the blood cholesterol.

Atheroma

It is unlikely that atheroma is a direct cause of hypertension but it is certain that, when the two conditions coexist, the risks are greatly increased.

Family history

Hypertension runs in families and most hypertensive patients can think of a relative who has it. This is not just because it is a common condition. If both parents have hypertension, half their children will be affected. If one parent is affected, the risk is one in four.

Diabetes

Diabetes and hypertension is a common and particularly dangerous combination. The cause and effect equation is impossible to disentangle. Diabetes, hypertension, hyperlipidaemia, obesity, atheroma and renal disease are interdependent.

It is these interwoven and mutually destructive relationships which make the combination of the two conditions so lethal.

Patients with any of these features in addition to hypertension need to be treated with the greatest enthusiasm.

Effects of hypertension

Target organs

Hypertension has effects on the heart itself and on the peripheral or target organs; especially the aorta, brain and kidneys. It accelerates the development of atheroma, and arterioles throughout the body are damaged although the precise impact on each tissue depends on its sensitivity to vascular changes.

The heart

The main effect on the heart is left ventricular hypertrophy. This is similar to the hypertrophy occurring in any muscle which is used excessively but it is an inconsistent process and the degree of hypertrophy in different individuals does not always match the degree of hypertension or the length of time it has been present. It appears that, in some people, hypertension may be associated with a sort of hypertrophic cardiomyopathy which results in hypertrophy out of all proportion to the levels of blood pressure recorded. It may be that, in these individuals, high alcohol intake is a significant contributory factor.

The hypertrophied muscle requires an increased blood supply. If this is not available because of ischaemic heart disease, then angina, myocardial infarction and heart failure, due to ischaemic damage (fibrosis), are likely.

Hypertensive patients with left ventricular hypertrophy have a worse prognosis than those without. The risk of myocardial infarction is four times as great, and that of stroke twelve times.

The arteries

Raised blood pressure is maintained by arteriolar vasoconstriction which causes increased peripheral resistance. This leads to hypertrophy of the arteriolar wall.

The effects of long-standing hypertension on large to medium-sized arteries are thickening of the vessel wall, endothelial damage and increased formation of atheroma (Figure 3.2). The compliance and elastic recoil of the vessels is reduced, leading to increased pulse pressure.

In the coronary arteries, this makes thrombosis and occlusion more likely (Figure 3.3).

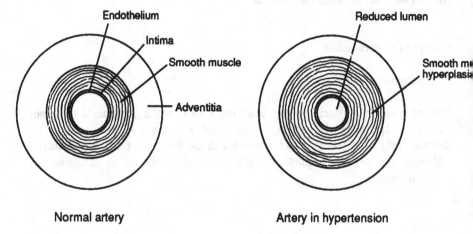

Normal artery   Artery in hypertension

Figure 3.2 Thickening of artery in hypertension

Degeneration of the intimal layers of the aorta is a normal part of ageing. If the blood pressure is raised, in the presence of damaged intima, the likelihood of dissection of the aorta is greatly increased.

The aorta becomes dilated during prolonged hypertension, making the development of aortic aneurysm more likely.

The brain

The effect of hypertension on the brain can be insidious or cataclysmic. Aneurysms form in the damaged arterioles and are liable to rupture causing cerebral haemorrhage. For this reason, subarachnoid haemorrhage is also more common in hypertensives.

Intimal damage and atheroma cause thromboses in small arteries and infarction of brain tissue.

It can also cause gradual, progressive deterioration of function with dementia.

Very severe hypertension can cause hypertensive encephalopathy, when the intracranial pressure rises and the patient loses consciousness. Death follows rapidly unless prompt treatment is given.

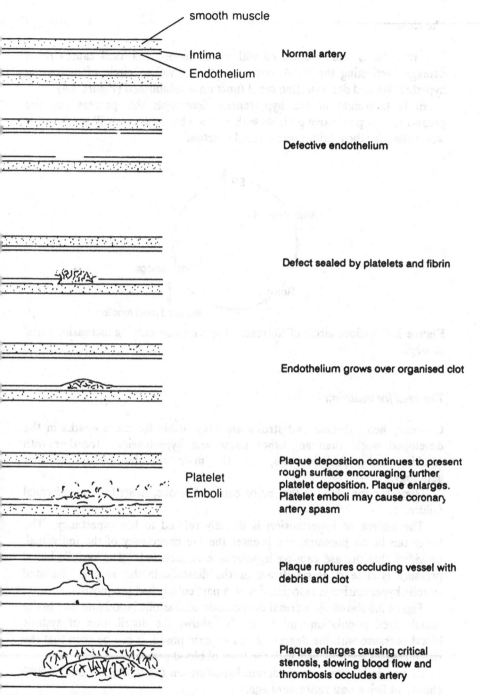

Figure 3.3 Atheromatous plaque formation

The kidneys

Hypertension is often associated with renal disease and itself causes renal damage, activating the RAA system so that a vicious circle of increasing hypertension and deteriorating renal function is established (Figure 3.4).

Early treatment of the hypertension interrupts this process but the prognosis of hypertensive patients with a raised blood urea is still significantly worse than for those with normal renal function.

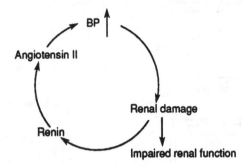

Figure 3.4 Vicious circle of untreated hypertension causing increasing renal damage

The need for treatment

Coronary heart disease and stroke are responsible for more deaths in the developed world than any other cause and hypertension, together with smoking and hyperlipidaemia, are the main alterable factors in their aetiology.

Hypertension alone is the major cause of stroke, heart failure and renal failure.

The degree of hypertension is directly related to life expectancy. The lower the blood pressure, the greater the life expectancy of the individual, provided that disease causing hypotension is excluded. The systolic blood pressure is at least as significant as the diastolic in this respect. Isolated systolic hypertension is associated with a particularly bad prognosis.

Figure 3.6 shows the normal distribution of diastolic blood pressure in the middle-aged population and Figure 3.7 shows the distribution of systolic blood pressure with the degree of risk superimposed. It can be seen that the risk increases continuously with the level of blood pressure.

A man in his 30s with moderate hypertension (150/100) has only a 50% chance of living past retirement age.

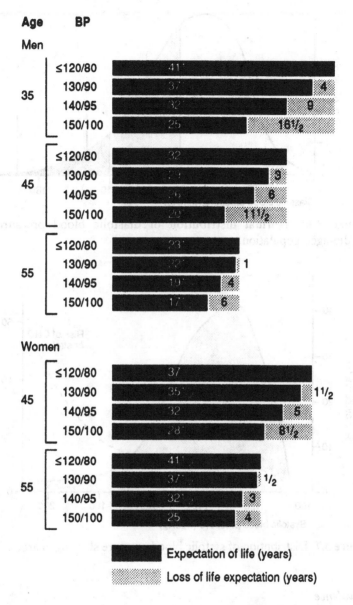

Figure 3.5 Correlation of life expectancy and blood pressure

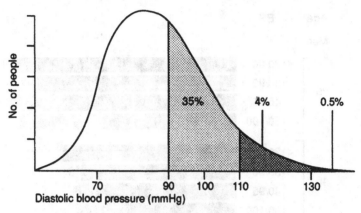

Figure 3.6 Normal distribution of diastolic blood pressure in the middle-aged population

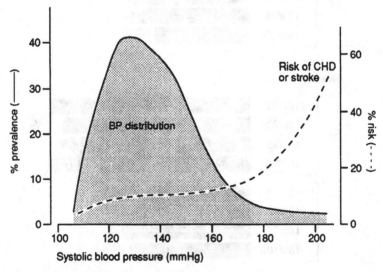

Figure 3.7 Distribution of systolic blood pressure showing degree of risk

Prevalence

Severe hypertension (systolic 130 + age; diastolic 110) affects about 5% of the adult population: 70–80 patients in an average GPs list.

A further 20% have mild to moderate hypertension: systolic pressure 120–130 + age and diastolic 90–109.

This means that a practice with 4 or 5 partners and 8000–9000 patients can expect to have up to 1500 patients with hypertension, all of whom need diagnosis and non-drug treatment and about half of whom will probably benefit from treatment with drugs.

At the present time, it is unlikely that more than a quarter of these are well controlled. The so-called 'rule of halves' has been coined to describe this situation:

Of 800 people with hypertension:
½ (400) are known;
½ of these (200) are treated;
½ of these (100) are well-controlled

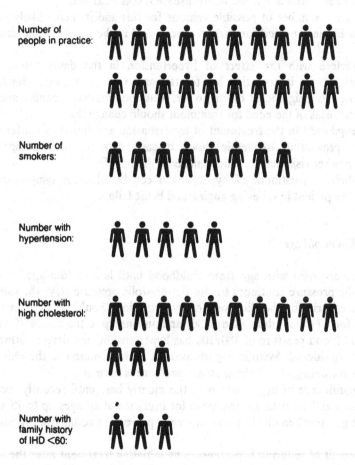

Figure 3.8 Incidence of risk factors in UK

The evidence that treating hypertension prevents death and disability resulting from stroke, heart failure, renal failure and dissection of the aorta is clear and the importance of screening for and treating confirmed hypertension is therefore well established.

However, the risks are not abolished altogether by treatment and it is important to realise that most patients who sustain cerebrovascular accidents or myocardial infarcts have only mild hypertension or blood pressure, which is average for their age. It is therefore of the greatest importance to treat other risk factors such as smoking and hyperlipidaemia as well as hypertension.

The evidence for the benefits of treating hypertension in relation to preventing death from ischaemic heart disease is less clear cut.

There are a number of possible reasons for this and it seems likely that the answer lies in the need for early diagnosis and in the effects of the drugs used.

To interfere with the effect of hypertension in the development of coronary atheroma, intervention has to start at a very early stage. This has not happened to a significant extent so far. Mass population screening and a greater awareness of the need for treatment should change this.

The drugs used in the treatment of hypertension and found to confer no benefit in preventing ischaemic heart disease may be introducing or aggravating other risk factors, which outweigh the benefits.

Nevertheless, treatment of hypertension can be of great symptomatic benefit to the patient in relieving angina and heart failure.

Hypertension in old age

Blood pressure rises with age from childhood until late middle age. After that, systolic pressure continues to rise but diastolic pressure stays the same. The same criteria for the diagnosis of hypertension should be used in the elderly as for all other adults (see p. 36) and anyone up to the age of 75 with a persistent blood pressure of 180/100 has hypertension, and drug treatment should be considered. Systolic hypertension is more common in the elderly and is worth treating even if the diastolic pressure is normal.

The significance of hypertension in the elderly has, until recently, been underestimated. The risks are the same for everyone at all ages up to 75 and in fact the greatest benefits in terms of stroke prevention result from treating the elderly.

The benefit of reducing hypertension by initiating treatment after the age of 75 years is more difficult to demonstrate. However, most doctors would not use a fixed figure for the upper age limit and would take into account the degree of overall fitness as an additional factor.

Patients over the age of 75 who are already taking hypotensive medication need particularly careful monitoring because of the risks of renal impairment, the need to reduce dose with increasing age and the risks of hypotension (see Chapter 8).

4

Diagnosis and assessment of essential hypertension

The setting for the management of hypertension

The cause of hypertension is multifactorial and its management in the population has several facets:

* screening
* confirmation of diagnosis
* assessment
* health education
* non-drug treatment
* drug treatment
* long-term monitoring

Since hypertension occurs randomly in all sections of the population and is common and asymptomatic at the stage diagnosis is needed, selective screening is inappropriate. Whole population screening is the only effective way of identifying hypertensive patients.

The diagnosis is complex and requires several consultations; borderline cases need long-term monitoring; these and many mild hypertensives need long-term, supervised non-drug treatment and those taking drug treatment also need careful long-term monitoring.

Health education of individuals at risk and of the population as a whole is an important part of the management. Good clinical care is useless without sound management to organise case finding and long-term monitoring.

Several related disciplines have to be involved in all this activity (Figure 4.1).

The only place that this level and complexity of care can happen in the UK is in General Practice, with its access to the entire population, the grouping of skilled personnel into primary health care teams and the increasing access to computers.

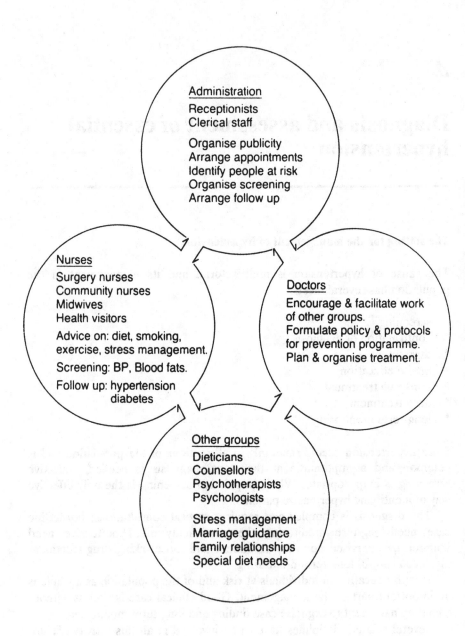

Figure 4.1 Groups involved in prevention

Screening

Patients with hypertension are usually symptomless and are identified only by screening or if the blood pressure is taken for another reason such as a routine examination for insurance or employment purposes, or when the patient is admitted to hospital or seen in an accident and emergency or outpatient department.

The diagnosis of hypertension cannot be made on the basis of one initial reading and further measurements at intervals are needed to confirm the diagnosis.

There is no way of knowing who may be suffering from hypertension and so to be effective, population screening has to be comprehensive. It is sensible to combine the measurement of blood pressure with health education and with other screening procedures, such as cervical smears, at the same appointment.

Most practices now run health promotion clinics for this purpose but it will never be possible to include every patient registered with the practice in clinics and it is important that those who do not attend a clinic do not get left out of the screening process.

It does not matter who takes the blood pressure provided they have had appropriate training and experience and use a protocol agreed by everyone in the practice (see below under diagnostic criteria).

The simplest way to make sure everyone's blood pressure is taken regularly every 3 years is to have a computer record incorporating a recall date.

The blood pressure is entered on the patient's computer record either by going through all records by hand or by waiting until he or she next attends.

If no computer is available, then a box of index cards can be used, one for each patient, divided into monthly sections. For 3-yearly checks, 36 dividers would be needed, one for each month of the 3 years. When a patient attends for a test, the card is placed in the section for the month after the next test is due. This allows for him to come late without being sent a reminder. At the end of each month, any cards remaining are extracted and the records checked to see if the test has in fact been done. If not, then a reminder is sent and the card placed in the next section.

This system works well for follow up of patients with long-term diseases such as asthma but is too cumbersome for mass screening for all but the smallest practices.

Some computer systems enable the receptionist to prepare an appointments list for each doctor with details of those screening or immunisation procedures which are due.

Alternatively, the notes of patients who are due for a blood pressure check can be tagged with a coloured marker as a reminder to the doctor.

These reminders can be ignored if the doctor is short of time or the patient is ill or unwilling to have the test. They will reappear next time the patient attends.

When a screening system is set up, as many as possible of those who are to be involved should be included in the planning. This means at least the practice manager, a receptionist, a practice nurse and a doctor. In this way some of the possible difficulties can be anticipated and avoided.

If the blood pressure is taken opportunistically, over 90% of the population can be screened every 3 years leaving only 10% to be chased up. This remaining 10% can cause real problems.

The results of postal letters of invitation are very poor with over half failing to attend. Telephone calls or home visits are slightly more effective but time-consuming and intrusive.

A major problem, especially in inner cities, is the mobility of the population.

A frequent reason for non-attendance is that the patient has had a blood pressure test somewhere else recently.

Blood pressure is often measured in the course of an episode or procedure which itself has nothing to do with screening for hypertension. Admission to hospital, a visit to an A & E department after an injury, an employment or insurance medical are common events. It would be immensely helpful if these readings could be reported to the patient's doctor.

It is tempting not to bother with those who fail to attend after repeated attempts to contact them. The worrying aspect of this is that this group may include some of the most vulnerable members of the community as cardiovascular disease bears hardest on the lower social classes, who are the least likely to respond to offers of health checks. Posters in social security offices and offers of health checks by employers may help to overcome this problem.

Medical records

Medical records must be well organised. Few practices have given up paper records altogether and even those that have need to make sure that the computer record is tidy and easily accessible if recordings of blood pressure are to be immediately available to anyone opening the file.

A separate summary sheet for all basic data is helpful (Figure 4.2).

If there is no summary sheet, it is difficult to keep track of dates and results of readings. Borderline readings may be overlooked and normal readings may be repeated unnecessarily.

If the last record of the blood pressure is immediately obvious to the doctor or nurse opening the notes, they are more likely to repeat it when the next reading is due. This reduces the number of people for whom special appointments have to be sent by letter.

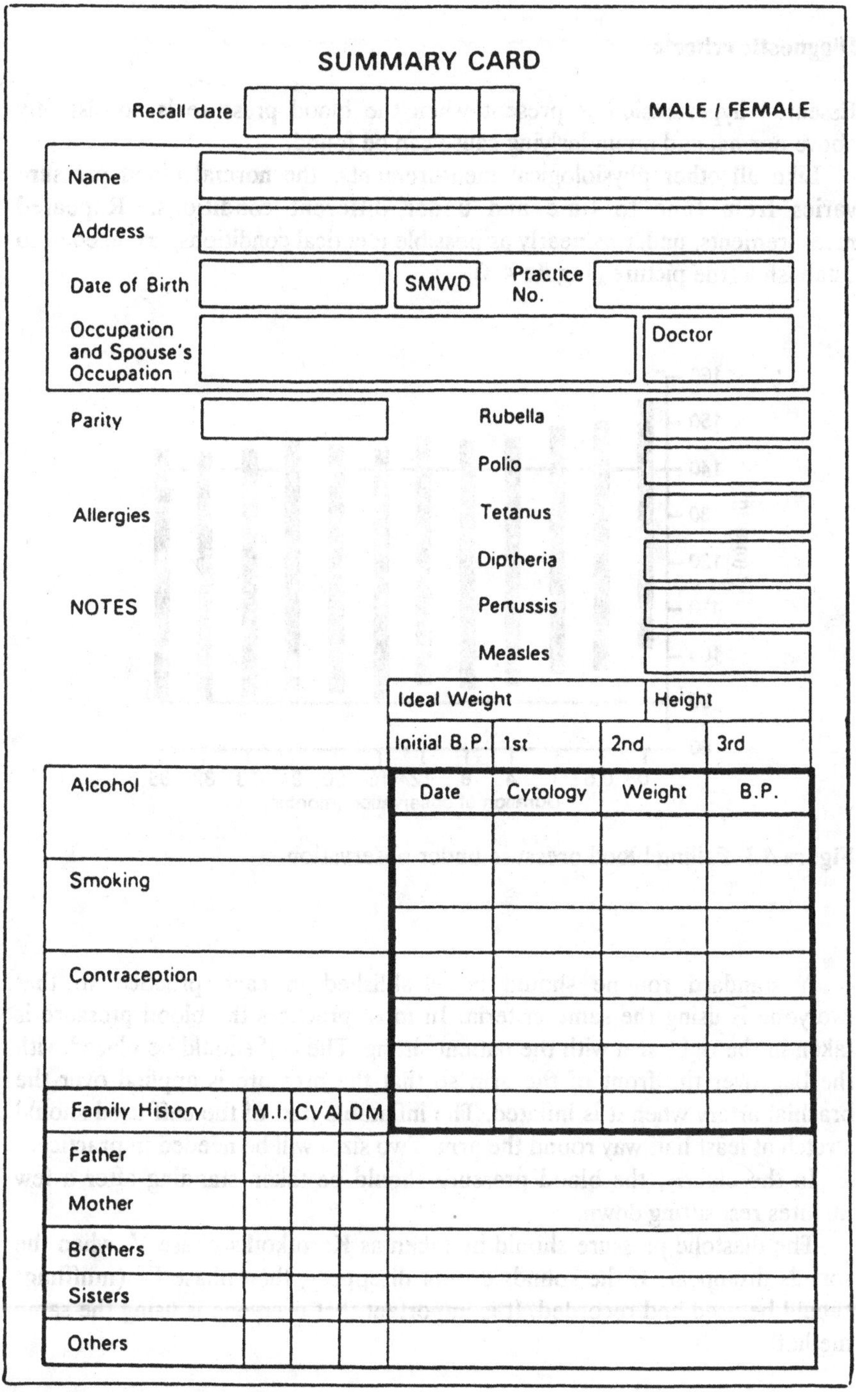

SUMMARY CARD

Recall date ☐☐☐☐☐☐   MALE / FEMALE

Name	
Address	

| Date of Birth | | SMWD | Practice No. | |

| Occupation and Spouse's Occupation | | Doctor |

Parity		Rubella	
		Polio	
Allergies		Tetanus	
		Diptheria	
NOTES		Pertussis	
		Measles	

| Ideal Weight | | Height | |
| Initial B.P. | 1st | 2nd | 3rd |

Alcohol		Date	Cytology	Weight	B.P.
Smoking					
Contraception					

Family History	M.I.	CVA	DM				
Father							
Mother							
Brothers							
Sisters							
Others							

Figure 4.2 Summary sheet

Diagnostic criteria

Essential hypertension is present when the blood pressure is consistently above normal and no underlying cause can be found.

Like all other physiological measurements, the normal blood pressure varies from time to time and under different conditions. Repeated measurements, under as nearly as possible identical conditions, are needed to establish a true picture (Figure 4.3).

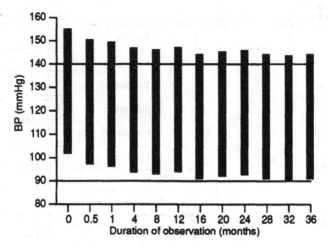

Figure 4.3 Falling blood pressure under observation

A standard routine should be established in each practice so that everyone is using the same criteria. In most practices the blood pressure is taken in the right arm with the patient sitting. The cuff should be placed with the bag over the front of the arm so that the pressure is applied over the brachial artery when it is inflated. The inflatable part of the cuff used should stretch at least half way round the arm. Two sizes will be needed in practice.

In the elderly, the blood pressure should be taken standing after a few minutes rest sitting down.

The diastolic pressure should be taken as Korotkoff's phase V, when the sounds disappear. If the sounds do not disappear, then phase IV (muffling) should be used and recorded. It is important that everyone is using the same method.

A useful, if rough, working definition of the upper limit of normal is:

Systolic: 100 + age

Diastolic: 90 for people under 50
            100 for people aged 50–70
            110 for people aged over 70

It is only if the pressure is consistently raised that the patient can be said to have hypertension.

Hypertension may be defined as follows:

	Systolic	Diastolic (5th phase)		
		< 50 y	< 50–70 y	> 70 y
Mild	> 100 + age	90–100	100–110	110–120
Moderate	> 120 + age	100–110	110–120	120–130
Severe	> 130 + age	> 110	> 120	> 130

Assessment

The diagnosis of hypertension should be based on a minimum of three readings taken on different occasions. At least six readings should be taken before drug treatment is started. This is essential because, however high the first reading, subsequent ones are nearly always lower and there is a danger of attributing the fall to treatment if a series of readings have not been taken at the outset.

If the readings are persistently high, it is necessary to discover whether the patient is suffering from benign essential hypertension or whether the hypertension is secondary to another condition. If other causes are excluded, it is important to discover the degree of target organ damage and to identify the presence of complicating conditions. The history, examination and investigations are designed to do this.

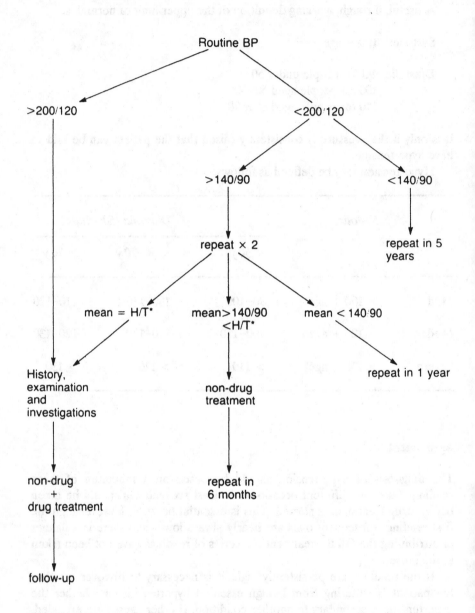

Figure 4.4 Protocol for hypertension screening
* depends on age

Conditions causing secondary hypertension:

* coarctation of the aorta (delayed femoral pulses, normal blood pressure in legs, rib notching on CXR);
* renal disease (proteinuria);
* Conn's syndrome (primary aldosteronism: low serum potassium);
* Cushing's syndrome (appearance, raised serum sodium and cortisol);
* phaeochromocytoma (very rare: intermittent symptoms, raised VMA)

Conditions and factors which may complicate hypertension:

* diabetes
* ischaemic heart disease
* peripheral vascular disease
* asthma
* stress factors
* smoking
* alcohol

History

This may provide clues to an underlying cause of the hypertension and forms the basis of the changes in life-style necessary for the non-drug treatment of the condition.

It will also be important if drug treatment is considered in future.

It may be useful to have a printed check list, which will be available in the notes for anyone who subsequently sees the patient.

* family history of H/T, IHD or CVA under age 60
* smoking
* alcohol consumption
* previous normal BP reading
* stress level/personality type
* asthma
* myocardial infarct
* CVA/TIA
* ureteric colic, pyelitis, haematuria
* chest pain
* breathlessness, cough
* intermittent claudication, Raynaud's phenomenon
* gout
* drugs

Examination

General appearance:

* build, weight, complexion (plethoric?);
* evidence of Cushing's syndrome, hyper- or hypothyroidism, anxiety, smoking, alcoholism, dementia;
* signs of hyperlipidaemia: arcus senilis, xanthelasma, tendon xanthomata.

Cardiovascular system:

* peripheral pulses including carotids
  – are femoral pulses delayed?

* Optic fundi (dilate the pupils if necessary):

  – Grade I: arterial thickening (silver wiring);
  – Grade II: arterial thickening, tortuosity and A–V nipping;
  – Grade III: haemorrhages and exudates;
  – Grade IV: papilloedema as well as Grade III changes.

* Heart:
  – check cardiac impulse for evidence of enlarged left ventricle
  – listen for aortic diastolic murmur of aortic regurgitation, especially if the hypertension is systolic with a wide pulse pressure.

Investigations

Although these are usually normal, they are important to exclude other causes, assess target organ damage and identify complicating conditions. They also form a baseline for the future.

* urine for protein, glucose, cells, casts and culture;
* blood for FBC, urea and electrolytes, sugar and cholesterol;

RESULT		POSSIBLE CAUSE
URINE:	Protein or blood	Renal disease
	Casts	Nephritis
	Glucose	Diabetes
BLOOD:	Urea ↑ ⎫ Creatinine ↑ ⎬	Renal failure; dehydration

K$^+$ <3.4 mmol/L	Diuretics; Conn's syndrome
Cholesterol ↑	Risk IHD ↑
Glucose >11.1 mmol/L	Diabetes mellitus
Uric acid ↑	Gout

ECG: May show evidence of previous infarction or ischaemia. Severe, long-standing hypertension always causes left ventricular hypertrophy (LVH) eventually. Some people develop LVH at an early stage. They have a worse prognosis and should be treated more vigorously.

ECG signs of LVH include:

- S in V1 + R in V6 = 40 mm (40 small squares) or more;
- S–T segment changes and T wave inversion in leads I, II, and V3–6. See Figure 4.5.

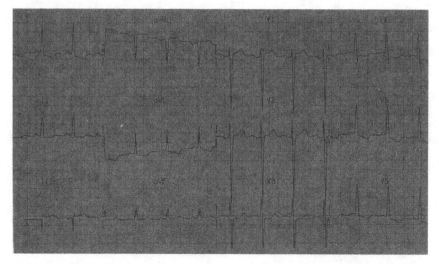

Figure 4.5 Left ventricular hypertrophy (National Medical Slide Bank)

* Chest X-ray to ascertain heart size, presence of dilatation of the aorta, rib notching, evidence of LVF.

* IVP if there is a history of renal disease.

5

The management of patients with hypertension

Health education

Health education is of the utmost importance.

None of the life-style changes necessary to reduce the incidence of hypertension and improve the outlook of patients with hypertension will happen without both a background of community-based health education and personally targetted advice.

Health education for the population as a whole comes mainly through the media but there are other routes from antenatal classes through playgroups and schools to local community groups, retirement courses and over-60s clubs. The messages have to be very powerful if they are to have an impact in the face of the promotion of cigarettes and alcohol.

District health authorities have a clear responsibility in this area but it is discharged erratically and they may need to be reminded of it from time to time.

Doctors and nurses can contribute to the process by making themselves available to local radio and groups to talk about risk factors and healthy life-styles.

In surgeries and health centres, posters and leaflets, videos and tapes all have a place.

Patients who have been identified as being at risk of cardiovascular disease or who have already been diagnosed can be helped both individually and in groups.

Health education in relation to cardiovascular disease should include smoking, exercise, diet, weight control and stress management.

Smoking

Smoking is a very important factor. There is little point in treating hypertension or hyperlipidaemia with expensive drugs if the patient sabotages the treatment by continuing to smoke. A statement to this effect can have a powerful impact and start the process of giving up.

The campaign against smoking starts with pregnancy and continues throughout life. Pre-conceptual counselling may be especially effective as parents are receptive at this point in their lives. Women and their partners should be non-smokers before conception. Ante-natal advice about smoking should continue throughout pregnancy if necessary. It is never too late to stop.

Passive smoking affects everyone, and children brought up with smokers are more likely to smoke themselves from an early age. Pregnant women and children should all live in non-smoking households so that any campaign should include all members of a household.

How best to help individual smokers to stop is the responsibility of every member of the primary health care team but the patient must not feel hounded. The smoker needs sympathy, support and encouragement as well as the fear of God and general disapproval. Doctors, health visitors, midwives, practice nurses and health education officers all have a part to play (Figure 5.1).

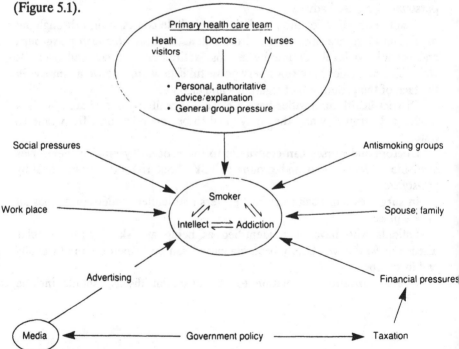

Figure 5.1 Help for smokers

44

Healthy diet

Unhealthy blood fats are important risk factors for coronary artery disease (see p. 13) but they are difficult to alter. This is mainly because they are determined not only by diet but by other factors.

Some individuals have an inherited tendency to high triglyceride and LDL levels. This can be exacerbated by an unhealthy life-style and if they are also hypertensive, their risks are multiplied.

Smoking and high stress levels appear to have an adverse effect on the ratio of HDL to LDL.

Men and post-menopausal women have less favourable HDL to LDL ratios than do pre-menopausal women.

High blood cholesterol levels can be improved to some extent by modifications in diet, and in the obese and those on very unhealthy diets, the effect can be dramatic. A cholesterol-lowering diet should be advised in all patients with hypertension or any other risk factor for cardiovascular disease even if the blood cholesterol is not grossly raised.

The main thrust of the diet should be to reduce saturated fats, increase the intake of oily fish, which has a protective effect, and maintain target weight (body-mass index) (Figure 5.2).

The greatest benefit of changes in diet result from its impact on children and in view of the familial nature of cardiovascular disease, dietary changes for adult patients should be for the whole family.

Exercise provides an increased feeling of fitness and sense of well-being, reduces stress levels, lowers blood pressure, improves the HDL/LDL ratio and helps in maintaining correct weight.

A healthy diet

A healthy diet should contain:

1. Plenty of:
    Vegetables, including potatoes, rice, pulses
    Fruit, including bananas
    Cereals, including bread
    Fish of all kinds, but especially oily fish

2. Moderate amounts (or none) of:
    Milk (skimmed for adults)
    Polyunsaturated fats, e.g. margarine
    Lean meat, offal, poultry
    Cheese (max. 8 oz per week full cream cheese like Cheddar)
    Eggs (max. three per week, including those in cooking)
    Salt

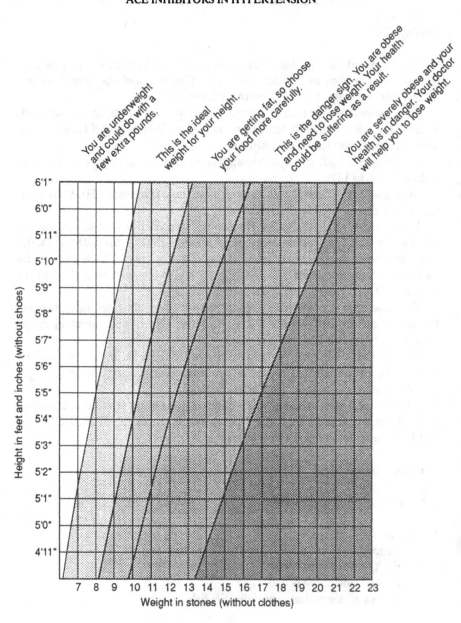

Figure 5.2 Height–weight chart showing risks

3. None of these:
   Dairy fats: cream, butter, full cream milk
   Crisps or chips (unless cooked in 'safe' oil, e.g. sunflower or corn oil)
   Sausages, burgers, fat minced meat
   Sugar or prepared foods with added sugar, e.g. most tinned fruit and soups

4. Only sunflower, maize or olive oil should be used in cooking

Treatment

More than in any other condition, the successful management of hypertension depends on a partnership between the patient, the doctor and other members of the primary health care team. No advice will be followed, or drugs taken, if the patient does not accept the need for treatment. The doctor may think he is treating the patient but in reality it is the patient who treats, or fails to treat, himself with help and advice from the doctor and the rest of the team.

There are several reasons why it is especially difficult for patients with hypertension to cooperate with treatment:

1. They have no symptoms and so no immediate benefit can be identified.

2. Changes in life-style are resented and seen as interfering with social life.

3. Treatment often needs to start when the patient is quite young and the theoretical threat of some distant disaster, such as a stroke, seems very far off and unreal.

4. Side-effects, both real and imagined, are common, especially during the early stages of treatment.

5. Visits to the surgery for blood pressure checks and adjustments to treatment have to be frequent at first and may seem very irksome.

6. Young people, who feel fit, do not like to be constantly reminded that there is something wrong with them. Taking medication reminds them every day.

7. Drug treatment in general gets a bad press from time to time and many people are understandably suspicious of it.

Once the diagnosis has been confirmed, the initial interview with the doctor is of crucial importance. The future success of the treatment depends on it. The doctor needs to know as much from the patient as the patient from the doctor. The details will depend on the individual, on how much is needed in the way of life-style changes and on whether the management is planned to include drugs.

The doctor needs to know what the patient already knows, or fears, about the condition and its treatment; whether he has any relatives or friends with hypertension and what their experience has been; what he feels about losing weight, giving up smoking and alcohol and taking exercise; how well he can be expected to cope with taking regular medication and any other individual considerations resulting from his work or interests.

The patient may not think of all his questions at once and it may be useful to anticipate his need for information, perhaps with a written advice leaflet.

He needs to know what hypertension is; how bad his is; what will happen if he has no treatment; what is the treatment and what it will achieve; how long he will have to continue to take it; whether it has any side-effects and what they are; how often he will have to come for check-ups; whether it will affect his work or prospects or his children.

It should be made clear that the decision to start treatment is the patient's. There is a choice. Most people are unable to take in all the information and implications at once and it is useful to allow time for consideration and delay starting until he has thought it over.

Non-drug treatment

The success of this depends on the persuasive skills of the doctor and practice nurse and the enthusiastic cooperation of the patient. It involves a life-long commitment to:

* non-smoking
* maintenance of correct weight
* regular exercise
* relaxation and stress management
* healthy diet

These are good general principles for a healthy life-style and should involve the whole family. They should be especially recommended to anyone with:

* a family history of hypertension
* occasional high blood pressure readings
* blood pressure at the upper end of the normal range
* confirmed hypertension, ischaemic heart disease, or diabetes

A low salt diet is worth trying for a few months. It may make a significant difference and make drug treatment unnecessary.

Certain drugs aggravate or cause hypertension in susceptible individuals. They include oral contraceptives, hormone replacement therapy, NSAIDs and systemic steroids. These should be avoided if possible in patients with hypertension and in those who have been found to have occasional high readings.

Even for those who are clearly going to need drug treatment, these general measures are important and can make a significant difference to the prognosis. Once drug treatment is started, there is a temptation to give them up. It is therefore helpful to get them well established before starting drugs.

Non-drug treatment should be given to all hypertensive patients for 2–3 months before drug treatment is started. During this time the investigations are carried out and further readings of the blood pressure are taken to establish a base line. It also allows time for the patient to get used to the diagnosis and for transient problems to pass.

In mild hypertension this may be all that is needed, especially if the patient had a large number of life-style changes to make and made them. If he or she is already a lean, active, relaxed, teetotal, non-smoker, then non-drug treatment will make little difference.

Drug treatment

Mild hypertension

The decision as to whether to prescribe drugs for patients with mild hypertension is not clear cut.

Women with mild hypertension benefit very little from drug treatment. If drugs are prescribed, it is better to avoid thiazide diuretics on their own.

Non-smoking men do benefit but the advantages can easily be outweighed by side-effects, lack of enthusiasm or poor compliance.

In smokers, the incidence of stroke is reduced by thiazides but not by β-blockers.

As a rough guide, drug treatment should be considered in:
* men or women:
    those with a diastolic pressure consistently over 100 mmHg;
* men alone:
    those with other risk factors such as diabetes, hyperlipidaemia, a family history of IHD or CVA under 60 years;
* anyone who has already sustained target organ damage:
    left ventricle: hypertrophy or failure;
    brain: stroke or encephalopathy;
    kidneys: impaired renal function.

Moderate and severe hypertension

All drug treatment should be combined with non-drug treatment as outlined above. This improves the efficacy of the drugs and allows the dose to be kept to a minimum.

The drugs commonly used are:

* Thiazide diuretics
* β-Blockers
* ACE inhibitors
* Calcium-channel blockers
* Peripheral vasodilators: hydralazine; α-blockers
* Methyldopa

There are a large number of preparations of these drugs available and strengths, side-effects, interactions and dosage regimes vary between the members of each group. Prescribing can be confusing and even dangerous if an attempt is made to use them all.

Every doctor should try to become familiar with one or two drugs from each group, usually prescribing from a short list of not more than ten. It is helpful if all the partners in a practice can agree on the short list so that the total number of different preparations in use by a practice is kept to a minimum. This helps the local pharmacist and dispensing practices to keep adequate but not excessive stocks.

Stepped care, in which treatment is started with a single drug and others are added in stages, has advantages over monotherapy. Better control is achieved because the drugs potentiate each other and the dose of each is kept to a minimum so that side effects and complications, which are dose-related, are reduced. About 80% of hypertensive patients are controlled by stepped care while under 50% are controlled by monotherapy. Initial treatment has often been diuretics or β-blocker but increased experience with newer drugs has widened our options and ACE inhibitors or calcium antagonists are now often used to start treatment. Stepped care must be governed by the patient's response; it should not become a standard treatment sequence.

Hypertension lends itself particularly well to the development of a practice management plan or protocol so that whoever sees the patient knows what is planned.

Table 5.1 Changes in BP and biochemical variables after 10 weeks' treatment with different doses of bendrofluazide

Mean change in:	Dose of bendrofluazide (mg per day)		
	2.5	5.0	10
Systolic BP (mmHg)	−14.3	−13.4	−17.0
Diastolic BP (mmHg)	−10.8	−10.1	−10.8
Potassium (mmol/L)	−0.20	−0.33	−0.45
Urate (μmol/L)	+29.0	+63.0	+68.0
Glucose (mmol/L)	+0.14	+0.04	+0.27
Cholesterol (mmol/L)	0.00	+0.02	+0.25

Before the drugs are chosen, an outline is needed so that both doctor and patient know what to expect. Here is an example:

* Allow 4 weeks between each visit.
* Check for side-effects at each visit.
* Aim for a diastolic pressure of 90 mmHg or less in a young and otherwise fit patient; between 90 and 100 mmHg in anyone who is elderly, frail or suffering from ischaemic heart disease.
* Continue to increase dose or add drugs until BP is controlled
* Avoid taking the blood pressure as soon as the patient sits down. A more reliable reading is obtained if the questioning comes first.

Drug plan

The most usual drug plan at the present time for an uncomplicated, non-smoking, hypertensive who is not diabetic or suffering from asthma, hyperlipidaemia or heart failure, might look like this:

Visit 1: β-Blocker e.g. atenolol 50 mg once daily.

Visit 2: Add bendrofluazide 2.5 mg once daily.

Visit 3: Add calcium-channel blocker, e.g. nifedipine tablets (not capsules) 10 mg twice daily. Note: there is no point in increasing the dose of β-blocker or diuretic.

Take blood pressure both sitting and standing from now on. Check blood urea and electrolytes now, when stabilised, after 3 months and then annually.

Visit 4: Increase nifedipine to 20 mg twice daily.

Visit 5: Increase nifedipine to 40 mg twice daily.

The regime is now:

1. Atenolol 50 mg tablets once daily
2. Bendrofluazide tablets 2.5 mg once daily
3. Nifedipine tablets 40 mg once daily

An ACE inhibitor can be used in place of the calcium channel blocker and, increasingly, ACE inhibitors will be the first line drugs of choice in many patients, particularly if the physician wants to avoid the adverse metabolic effects associated with diuretics and β-blockers (see Chapter 7).

If the blood pressure is still not controlled, the possibility of an underlying condition causing secondary hypertension should be reconsidered. If the diagnosis is still benign essential hypertension, then other drugs can be added to the regime or a new start made with a different regime. This and the treatment of the large group of patients for whom this regime is unsuitable from the outset will be discussed in Chapter 8.

Long-term monitoring

Whether or not drug treatment is used, long-term follow-up is very important as the severity of the condition and therefore the indications for treatment may change.

If the patient is not taking drugs, this may be done by the practice nurse as long as she or he has appropriate training and a protocol agreed by the whole primary health care team. The individual criteria for each patient should be written in the notes by the doctor. If the patient is taking hypotensive drugs, the follow-up can be shared between doctor and nurse.

A reliable recall system is essential. It is not enough to leave it to the patient to return at the recommended intervals. A computer recall system is the simplest method but if no computer is available, the index card system, described on page 33 for screening, can be used.

A long-term treatment protocol is a useful check list for follow-up as it means that the same system is being used, whoever sees the patient, and makes sure that important checks are not omitted due to pressure of work or time constraints. If a patient-held treatment card is included in the plan, information is immediately available to hospital staff if it is needed and the patient also knows what to expect and is more likely to share the enthusiasm of the practice for treating the disease.

Example of follow-up plan for hypertensive patients on drug treatment, 3 months after initial stabilisation:

Table 5.2

Seen by	Observations	Next appointment
Doctor	Compliance: drugs & non-drug treatment. Well-being; side-effects, symptoms. Blood pressure. Complete patient's card	3 months
Doctor	As above	3 months
Nurse	Weight, BP, well-being, worries, symptoms, test urine, take blood for U&Es, compliance, complete patient card.	6 months
Doctor	Annual check: examn. of CVS, fundi, ECG, urine, U&Es, symptoms, compliance, life-style. Reassess original indications for starting treatment, choice & dose of drugs. If BP well controlled, consider reducing drugs. Complete patient-held record card.	6 months

Thereafter the patient is seen alternately by the doctor and the nurse who uses the protocol in Table 5.3. Prescriptions for 3 months' supply of drugs are given at each visit with authorisation for one 3-month repeat prescription between visits.

Table 5.3 Guidelines for long-term follow-up of hypertensive patients by nurses

---

Ask about:
* well-being
* life-style: smoking, alcohol, exercise
* exercise tolerance
* symptoms: chest pain, breathlessness, leg pains

Check drugs: dose, compliance, side-effects, OTC drugs

Measure:
* weight
* BP sitting; standing if over 60 or taking vasodilator

Test urine

Take blood if due (see medical records)

Refer to doctor if symptomatic, BP outside agreed range (see medical records) or has missed appointment

Note results in medical record and in patient-held card

Discuss problems; advise life-style

Make next appointment

6

The ACE inhibitor drugs:
history and pharmacology

History of development

The workings of the renin–angiotensin system have been the subject of study for nearly a century. As long ago as 1898, Scandinavian researchers extracted a substance from the kidney which was found to exert a powerful pressor effect.

The nature of this substance was not elucidated until the 1930s when a number of scientists around the world developed animal models which enabled them to study hypertension. In these, the flow of blood to the kidney was reduced by artificial constriction of the renal artery. It was noticed that the kidney responded by generating a chemical substance that raised blood pressure, overcoming the resistance in the renal artery. When the artery was unclamped, blood pressure returned to normal.

The substance was subsequently identified as angiotensin, and in the 1950s further work established that it existed in two forms: angiotensin I and angiotensin II. An enzyme – angiotensin-converting enzyme – was responsible for the conversion of the inactive angiotensin I to the active angiotensin II hormone.

Meanwhile, independent research being conducted into the properties of snake venom was to provide a vital link between this basic research and the synthesis of a new class of antihypertensive agent.

In 1965, the venom of a Brazilian snake, *Bothrops jararaca*, was found to contain a substance that inhibited kininase II. Kininase II cleaves a dipeptide from the vasodilator bradykinin, destroying its vasodilating activity. The substance in the snake venom responsible for blocking this degradation, was appropriately named 'bradykinin-potentiating factor'. A decade later it was established that kininase II and angiotensin-converting enzyme were one and the same substance.

So the enzyme responsible for producing a powerful vasoconstrictor is also capable of breaking down a potent vasodilator.

The antihypertensive properties of the peptides in the snake venom were confirmed and a systematic search for therapeutic agents began. This culminated in 1977 with the development of the first ACE inhibitor, captopril, followed in 1980 by enalapril. There are now eight ACE inhibitors available for prescribing in this country and many more are in the research pipeline.

Early problems with ACE inhibitors

When captopril was first launched it was used in patients with complicated conditions including collagen vascular disease and severe renal disease. A failure to appreciate that dosage adjustments were required in patients with renal insufficiency occasionally led to acute hypotensive episodes and, on chronic dosing, to accumulation of the drug with evidence of toxicity. Cases of agranulocytosis and neutropenia caused particular alarm and ACE inhibitors came to be regarded as therapy of last resort. Initially, the unwanted effects were thought to be due to the presence of the sulphydryl group in captopril, spurring the development of ACE inhibitors without this group.

Eventually it was realised that the serious side effects were not due to chemical structure at all but could be avoided simply by limiting the daily dose. By this time the reputations of captopril and enalapril had been blighted by the early failure to assess a safe and effective dose and it took a number of years for the true side-effect profile to emerge.

The renin–angiotensin–aldosterone system (RAAS)

There is still a lot to be learnt about the way in which ACE inhibitors bring about a reduction in blood pressure, but the major mechanism involves de-activation of the RAA system, the physiology of which we will review briefly here.

Angiotensinogen is a large glycoprotein synthesized primarily in the liver but also found in other tissues such as the kidney and brain. Another glycoprotein, renin, cleaves one end of the angiotensinogen substrate to produce the physiologically inactive decapeptide angiotensin I. Renin is mainly synthesized by the juxtaglomerular cells in the media of the renal afferent arteriole but has also been found in other tissues including the brain, blood vessels, genital tract, adrenal glands and in tumours.

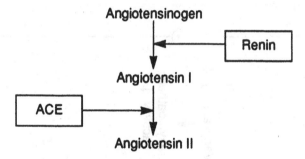

Figure 6.1 Site of action of enzymes

Angiotensin I is converted by ACE (angiotensin converting enzyme) to the physiologically active octapeptide, angiotensin II.

Angiotensin II

Angiotensin II is the most potent vasoconstrictor known, affecting the arterioles more than the veins, and the vessels in the skin and kidney more than those in muscle and the brain. It has many other effects, all of which contribute to the raising of blood pressure:

- It stimulates secretion of aldosterone, which acts at the distal nephron, increasing sodium and water retention, and increasing blood volume.
- It stimulates sympathetic activity causing vasoconstriction.
- It increases cardiac output (but not heart rate).
- It enhances ADH (vasopressin) secretion.
- It enhances corticotrophin (ACTH) secretion.
- It also has a number of renal effects:
  - It suppresses the release of renin via a negative feedback mechanism.
  - It causes vasoconstriction, mainly at the efferent arteriole.
  - It increases tubular sodium reabsorption.

Angiotensin II is eventually converted to the much less active angiotensin III by the action of aminopeptidase, and both forms are broken down to inactive fragments by angiotensinases distributed throughout the body.

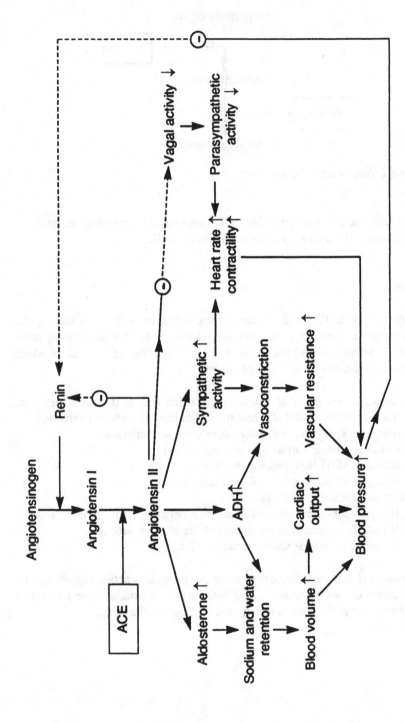

Figure 6.2 Actions of angiotensin II

Angiotensin-converting enzyme (ACE)

ACE is widely distributed in the body, and is found in high concentrations in the lung, kidneys, adrenals, brain and vascular and cardiac tissue. As well as promoting vasoconstriction by the formation of angiotensin II, it degrades the vasodilator bradykinin.

Function of the RAA system

The renin–angiotensin–aldosterone system is a sensitive physiological mechanism which helps to maintain blood pressure and blood volume. It responds to changes in the perfusion pressure of the kidney and to changes in blood volume by adjusting solute resorption and vascular tension. Renin appears to be the rate-limiting component of the system with release being stimulated by a number of factors:

- vascular stretch of the afferent arteriole of the glomerulus.
- electrolyte content (mainly Na^+) in the distal tubule which is sensed by the macula densa
- levels of angiotensin II through a negative feedback loop.

Anything which lowers renal perfusion pressure, such as reduced cardiac output, lowered total peripheral resistance, reduction in blood volume, will result in activation of the RAA system.The system serves the body well in coping with day-to-day physiological changes, but in the hypertensive individual the normal 'setting' of the system appears to be too high, with the consequence that blood pressure is maintained at an undesirably high level.

Mode of action of ACE inhibitors

Three actions of the ACE inhibitors are clinically significant:
- inhibition of angiotensin II production
- reduction of plasma aldosterone
- promotion of bradykinin activity.

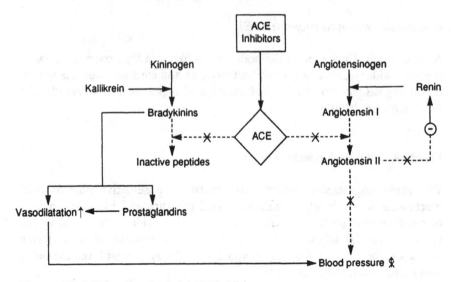

Figure 6.3 Mode of action of ACE inhibitors

Inhibition of angiotensin II production

The predominant clinical effect of ACE inhibitors is inhibition of angiotensin II synthesis. The immediate hypotensive response is therefore directly related to the pre-treatment levels of angiotensin II in plasma, and hence to pre-treatment plasma renin activity (PRA). However, during long-term use, ACE inhibitors control blood pressure in patients with low, as well as high, PRA. The possible explanation for this is discussed later. Renin levels rise as a result of the removal of negative feedback by angiotensin II. High levels of angiotensin I develop as conversion to angiotensin II is blocked.

Reduction of plasma aldosterone

ACE inhibitors cause a marked reduction in plasma aldosterone which reduces tubular resorption of water and salt, and increases tubular resorption of potassium.

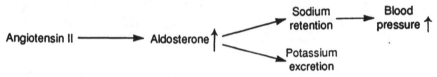

Figure 6.4 Actions of aldosterone

Potentiation of bradykinin activity

The RAA system is only one of the hormonal systems which regulate blood pressure: the kallikrein–kinin system and prostaglandins have vasodilator activity which may provide a physiological counterbalance to the vasopressor actions of angiotensin II. In addition to causing inhibition of ACE in serum and tissues, ACE inhibitors can potentiate the hypotensive activity of bradykinin. In turn, kinins can release vasodilating prostaglandins such as PGE2 from a variety of tissues. However, research into the precise role of kinins and prostaglandins in the action of ACE inhibitors has provided conflicting results and the situation is by no means completely understood.

Clinical effects

Reduction in blood pressure

In normal subjects and in hypertensive individuals without left ventricular failure, ACE inhibitors cause a decrease in blood pressure due to a decrease in systemic vascular resistance. Renal, splanchnic and liver vascular beds are more affected than skeletal muscle and brain vascular beds. Blood pressure is also reduced by a reduction in blood volume brought about by inhibition of ADH activity. The reduction in ADH activity also causes a decrease in thirst and salt appetite.

Cardiac effects

The decrease in blood pressure occurs without a significant change in cardiac output or heart rate, except in patients with congestive heart failure, where more marked increases in cardiac output have been seen. The fall in blood pressure does not bring about reflex tachycardia, probably because the vagal inhibition caused by angiotensin II is removed, and possibly because of a 'resetting' of baroreceptor sensitivity.

Renal effects

In spite of a decreased blood pressure, ACE inhibitors increase renal blood flow probably due to removal of the vasoconstricting effects of angiotensin II on the efferent arteriole. They have no marked effect on glomerular filtration in the normal kidney.

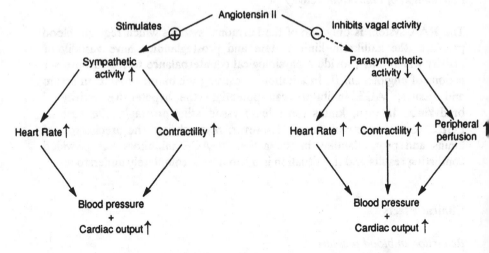

Figure 6.5 Influence of angiotensin II on the autonomic nervous system

When perfusion pressure is low, as in for instance, renal artery stenosis, glomerular filtration is maintained by vasoconstriction of the efferent arteriole. ACE inhibition may induce renal insufficiency by eliminating this vasoconstricting effect of angiotensin II and thereby reducing GFR.

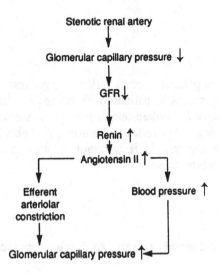

Figure 6.6 Renal artery stenosis and GFR

Changes in arterial wall structure

Chronic hypertension is associated with an increase in smooth muscle cell mass in the arterial walls, and an increase in the ratio of collagen to elastin. The vessels become rigid, dilated and weakened with a decrease in compliance. This diminishes their ability to buffer the fluctuations of arterial pressure during the normal cardiac cycle, resulting in increased pulse pressure.

Animal studies have demonstrated that ACE inhibitor treatment has a beneficial effect on arterial wall structure, decreasing arterial wall thickness and reversing smooth muscle cell hypertrophy. Improvements in the elastin:collagen ratio have also been noted. These changes have measurable effects on the arterial walls producing a noticeable improvement in vascular function in hypertensive patients.

Cardioprotection and cardiac hypertrophy

ACE inhibitors have been found to exert a cardioprotective effect: studies have shown that there are significant reductions in mortality in patients treated with enalapril (in addition to diuretics and digoxin) for moderate and severe congestive heart failure. Captopril has also exhibited cardioprotective effects.

Although left-ventricular hypertrophy is related to elevated blood pressure, agents which bring about a reduction in blood pressure do not necessarily reverse LVH. In this respect ACE inhibitors appear to be effective, and rapid reversal of left-ventricular hypertrophy in hypertensive patients has been demonstrated. It is suspected that angiotensin II reduces compliance of the large arteries, increasing the impedance to ventricular ejection and adding extra stress to the ventricular wall at the end of systole, which could contribute to left ventricular hypertrophy.

Endogenous RAA systems

It was initially thought that the main target of the ACE inhibitors was a circulating renin–angiotensin system but this could not fully explain a number of observations including:

- why ACE inhibitors were effective in patients with normal or low plasma renin activity (PRA)
- why the antihypertensive response lasted much longer than the duration of plasma ACE inhibition.

There is now substantial evidence for the existence – in addition to the endocrine RAAS – of endogenous renin–angiotensin systems in many tissues such as brain, heart, vascular tissue, kidney, gonads and intestine. In these, angiotensin II may exert an autocrine influence on the cells in which it is produced or a paracrine influence on adjacent cells. In fact the RAA system could be viewed as having two parts: a circulating part and another in local tissues. The circulating RAA system provides immediate cardiorenal homeostasis while the intrinsic system provides control of vascular resistance and local tissue function.

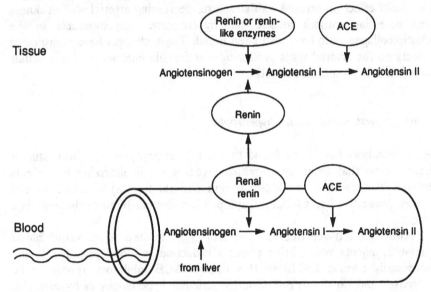

Figure 6.7 Inter-relationship between tissue and circulating renin–angio-tensin–aldosterone systems

The angiotensin converting enzyme (ACE), as a component of the local tissue RAAS, may differ slightly in various tissues and may bind ACE inhibitors to differing degrees. Thus, the potency of ACE inhibitors in inhibiting tissue ACE appears to vary; in heart and lung tissues, the order of potency is quinaprilat > perindoprilat > lisinopril > enalaprilat > fosino-prilat. Inhibition of tissue ACE may also explain why the effect of some ACE inhibitors lasts longer than would be expected from the blood levels; indeed, the most potent drug in the above series produces significant inhibition of ACE in lung, heart and kidney tissue when blood levels are undetectable.

Summary of clinical effects

Short-term

- peripheral vasodilatation
- reduced plasma volume
- fall in blood pressure
- improved renal function (except in patients with renal artery stenosis or sodium depletion)
- reduced serum sodium; slight increase in serum potassium

Long-term
- possible regression of vascular hypertrophy.
- improved cardiac output in patients with heart failure
- improved survival in patients with heart failure

Pharmacokinetics

All ACE inhibitors are absorbed after oral administration, but enalapril, quinapril, ramipril and perindopril are pro-drugs which are inactive until they have been metabolised in the liver. Lisinopril and captopril are supplied in the active form. Captopril is the most rapidly absorbed but also has the shortest half-life. The other preparations have elimination half-lives ranging from 25 to 35 hours which is reflected in a long duration of action. The half-life of quinaprilat (the active form of the drug) is 2 hours but its duration of action is 24 hours, suggesting that tissue ACE inhibition is important (see above).

Excretion of ACE inhibitors is primarily by the kidneys.

Plasma protein binding is variable between the agents, being about 30% for captopril, 50% for enalaprilat (the active form of enalapril) and insignificant in the case of lisinopril. Protein binding may have clinical significance when ACE inhibitors are administered with highly protein-bound drugs such as NSAIDs.

All the drugs are widely distributed in most tissues and much current research is being directed to establishing how individual drugs compare in their ability to penetrate various tissue types. This would be reflected in the pharmacodynamic profile and could possibly be exploited in the development of tissue-specific ACE inhibitors.

Pharmacodynamics

To date, no significant clinical differences have emerged between the eight currently-marketed ACE inhibitors. The differences that do exist are mainly seen in the pharmacodynamic profiles where rate of onset and duration of action reflect the pharmacokinetic properties of the different preparations.

	Time of onset	Maximum effect reached within	Duration of action
Captopril	15 minutes	30–60 minutes	3–4 hours
Enalapril	1–2 hours	4–8 hours	24 hours
Lisinopril	2–4 hours	6–8 hours	24 hours
Quinapril	1 hour	2–4 hours	24 hours
Perindopril	1 hour	4–6 hours	24 hours
Ramipril	1–2 hours	4–8 hours	24 hours

Indications

Hypertension

In hypertension, several ACE inhibitors (e.g. captopril, enalapril, lisinopril) are now available for use as initial treatment, whereas in the early days of these drugs they were restricted to use when standard therapy had failed. Similar extensions will probably be applied eventually to other ACE inhibitors. Traditionally, ACE inhibitors have been added to treatment regimes based on β-blockers or diuretics and could be used alone only if the patient had co-existing problems such as diabetes or asthma. As reports of their clinical effectiveness and safety profile grew they came to be regarded favourably as first-line therapy for many patients and this has been reflected by the changes in approved indications.

Heart failure

Captopril, enalapril, lisinopril and quinapril are all indicated as adjunct therapy for congestive heart failure. They have revolutionised the treatment of congestive heart failure and are now often used with diuretics as first-line therapy for acute as well as chronic failure.

ACE inhibitor therapy has the advantage of interrupting the vicious circle of congestive heart failure: reduced cardiac output leading to more resistance and hence leading to a further reduction in output.

Dosage information in hypertension

All ACE inhibitors except captopril can be given once-daily.

	Daily starting dose	Daily maintenance dose	Maximum daily dose
Captopril	6.25 mg	50–100 mg	150 mg
Enalapril	2.5 mg	10–20 mg	40 mg
Lisinopril	2.5 mg	10–20 mg	40 mg
Quinapril	5 mg	20–40 mg	80 mg
Perindopril	2 mg	4–8 mg	8 mg
Ramipril	1.25 mg	2.5–5 mg	10 mg

7

Safety and side-effects of ACE inhibitors

In this chapter we will review the safety profile of six of the currently-available ACE inhibitors, comparing them with other antihypertensive therapies.

Initial problems

ACE inhibitors are one of the few classes of drugs where adverse effects can be said to have diminished with clinical use.

When they were first introduced, very high doses were used and therapy was concentrated on particularly fragile patients. Serious adverse effects emerged and these, combined with the occasional death encountered during this period, resulted in their acquiring a very poor safety reputation.

But as more patients were treated, and as dosage regimes were shifted downwards, it became clear that serious adverse effects were rare occurrences, usually associated with high doses and patients with renal impairment, hepatic impairment or electrolyte imbalance.

Providing that appropriate precautions are observed with these patients, and that recommended dosage levels are followed, ACE inhibitors will provide effective therapy with fewer side-effects than are generally seen with other antihypertensive drugs.

Indeed ACE inhibitors have a very 'clean' profile compared with other therapies.

Comparison with other antihypertensive therapies

ACE inhibitors are free of the centrally-mediated effects, such as insomnia, fatigue, depression, hallucinations and exercise intolerance seen with β-blockers. β-Blockers bring about a rise in peripheral resistance, and a reduction in cardiac output and heart rate which increases the risk of heart failure.

Calcium antagonists are associated with tachycardia, flushing, headache and constipation: effects which are rarely serious but which can become intolerable, leading to termination of the treatment.

ACE inhibitors are also free from the unfavourable metabolic effects which are often noted with thiazide diuretics. These include hypokalaemia leading to arrhythmias, hyperuricaemia leading to gout, and glucose intolerance which may precipitate diabetes or lead to loss of control in established cases. Furthermore, they raise total cholesterol levels and reduce the HDL/total cholesterol ratio.

Side-effect profile

All ACE inhibitors produce some common side-effects such as first-dose hypotension, cough, rash and taste impairment. They must also be used with great care in volume-depleted patients, and those with renal or hepatic impairment.

Used in this way, the incidence of side-effects with ACE inhibitors in double-blind trials has been less than 10% and adverse effects have not been serious. This compares with rates of up to 20% with some β-blockers and diuretics.

The most commonly observed side-effects, seen with all ACE inhibitors, include:
- dry cough
- headache
- dizziness
- gastrointestinal disturbances (nausea, vomiting, abdominal pain, diarrhoea – often transient)
- raised serum creatinine
- raised blood urea nitrogen (BUN)
- taste impairment (dysgeusia – rare).

Cough

A dry cough, occurring in 5–10% of patients, is one of the more common side-effects. Hormonal and local mediators have been investigated but the reasons for the cough are still unclear.

It has been treated successfully with non-steroidal anti-inflammatory drugs, which suggests that prostaglandins may play a role. However, as NSAIDs antagonise the antihypertensive effect of ACE inhibitors, by causing sodium retention, they are not recommended as a means of treating the cough.

If it becomes intolerable an alternative antihypertensive therapy should be sought, as patients who cough with one ACE inhibitor will usually cough with all others.

Taste

Clinically, this side-effect may present as loss of hypertensive control as many patients will increase their salt intake when they begin to lose taste.

First-dose response

The first dose of an ACE inhibitor may occasionally cause a steep drop in blood pressure. This is more likely to occur in patients with secondary hypertension, high pre-treatment blood pressure or high PRA. The latter group includes those patients who have been receiving high-dose diuretic therapy, which activates the RAA system. In such cases it is usual to start ACE inhibitor therapy with a low dose taken before going to bed when the consequences of hypotension will be minimised.

Patients particularly at risk, such as the elderly or those with heart failure, are often admitted to hospital for the start of ACE inhibitor therapy. The maximum fall of blood pressure is related to the time of peak ACE inhibition and the most critical period can therefore be predicted with some accuracy.

An excessive fall in blood pressure should be treated with a head-down tilt and infusion of a plasma expander if necessary. In severe cases an infusion of angiotensin II can be given.

Using small doses at the initiation of therapy does not avoid the risk of hypotension, but the duration of the episode will be shorter.

First-dose hypotension does not preclude subsequent successful use of the drug in the same patient.

Angioneurotic oedema

This is a rare but life-threatening complication of ACE inhibitor therapy which usually occurs during the first month of treatment. There is an abrupt local increase of vascular permeability which allows fluid to leak from blood vessels into surrounding tissues. If swelling is severe, breathing may be impeded.

Milder hypersensitivity reactions include pruritus, rash and fever: these are usually reversible on termination of therapy.

Blood dyscrasias, bone marrow depression, agranulocytosis

These are rare reactions, which are observed mostly in patients with renal impairment, especially if they have collagen vascular disease.

Hyperkalaemia

Hyperkalaemia has been observed very rarely in hypertensive patients, and is associated with risk factors such as renal insufficiency, and use of potassium-sparing diuretics and potassium supplements.

Renal deterioration

This is a particular problem in pre-existing bilateral renal disease, but is usually reversible if it is recognised and treated early.

Precautions

Concomitant diuretic therapy

It is recommended that diuretic therapy be withdrawn before starting treatment with ACE inhibitors, to reduce the likelihood of hypotension. Diuretics bring about a reflex activation of the RAA system which is blocked by the concomitant use of ACE inhibitors leading, on occasion, to a precipitous drop in blood pressure. If required, diuretics can be added in again once ACE inhibitor therapy has been established.

Potassium-sparing diuretics should be avoided: if they are used, serum potassium levels should be monitored.

Certain groups of patients must be treated with caution: the elderly, those with renal impairment, hepatic impairment, heart failure or electrolyte imbalance. These groups will be discussed in more detail in the following chapter.

Elderly

Elderly patients often have impaired renal and hepatic function which may lead to accumulation of drugs. Reduced dosage and regular monitoring is usually recommended. There is also an increased risk of serious injury if hypotension should lead to a fall.

Renal impairment

In patients with hypertension due to renal artery stenosis, glomerular filtration pressure is maintained in the face of reduced renal perfusion by activation of the RAA system. Angiotensin II production causes vaso-constriction of the efferent glomerular arteriole, increasing glomerular perfusion pressure and enhancing filtration into the renal tubule.

Blockade of the RAA system by ACE inhibitors will cause the efferent arteriole to dilate, decreasing the glomerular filtration pressure and hence the GFR.

In patients with unilateral renal stenosis this is rarely a problem as the other kidney will usually accommodate the drop in flow. But in the rarer cases of bilateral renal artery stenosis, or where the patient has a single kidney, renal failure may occur.

In cases of pre-existing renal impairment renal function should be closely monitored.

Hepatic impairment

When administering an ACE inhibitor which exists as a pro-drug, the patient with hepatic impairment should be kept under close medical supervision. Metabolism of the pro-drugs takes place in the liver, with formation of the active compound being delayed in cases of hepatic impairment. This may result in elevated levels of the administered compound.

Heart failure

Hypertensive patients with heart failure, with or without associated renal insufficiency, may display symptomatic hypotension on treatment with ACE inhibitors. In these patients, therapy should be started under close medical supervision in hospital.

Contraindications

Hypersensitivity to the drug
History of angioneurotic oedema
Pregnancy
Children: Use in children has not yet been studied and is not recommended.

8
Special patient groups

Due to the presence of coexisting conditions, or to advancing age, certain groups of patients can be particularly at risk from the effects of hypertension. Although treatment is desirable, it is frequently complicated in that some antihypertensive therapies may not be recommended, or may even be contraindicated.

However, the wide choice of antihypertensive drugs available means that there are usually suitable alternatives should one therapy prove inappropriate.

It is the purpose of this chapter to highlight some of the groups of patients particularly at risk and to discuss the most appropriate therapy in each case.

Special patient groups

Coexisting cardiovascular conditions
- left ventricular hypertrophy
- congestive heart failure
- ischaemic heart disease
- hyperlipidaemia
- heart block
- peripheral vascular disease
Asthma
Diabetes mellitus
Renal failure
Elderly
Pregnancy

Left ventricular hypertrophy (LVH)

About 50% of patients with moderate hypertension (diastolic pressures between 110 and 120 mmHg) show some degree of LVH. The prognosis is poor as LVH is the major risk factor for cardiac failure and is also associated with an increased risk of angina, myocardial infarction and sudden death. This risk is not accounted for on the basis of blood pressure alone and regression of LVH is not an inevitable result of blood pressure control. As we shall see, not all drugs are equally effective in reducing left ventricular mass.

There is good evidence that propranolol, atenolol, metoprolol and timolol lead to a regression of LVH, probably because of their ability to slow heart rate. Pindolol, which does not slow heart rate, also does not cause a reduction in left ventricular mass.

Calcium antagonists such as diltiazem and nifedipine bring about peripheral vasodilatation with some reflex tachycardia.

ACE inhibitors have been found to be very effective at reducing left ventricular mass while providing good control of blood pressure.

Thiazide diuretics. There is some doubt about the ability of any diuretic to cause regression of LVH and trial results are conflicting.

Indapamide – a non-thiazide diuretic – has been clearly shown to cause a significant reduction in left ventricular mass while also reducing blood pressure.

Vasodilators cause no regression even though they control blood pressure well. This may be due to the reflex tachycardia which vasodilators commonly bring about.

In summary, agents such as vasodilators and thiazide diuretics which, despite good control of blood pressure, bring about abnormal haemodynamic changes, are generally ineffective in reversing LVH.

Drugs such as β-blockers, calcium antagonists and ACE inhibitors achieve regression because, in addition to controlling blood pressure, they remove the stimuli to hypertrophy.

Summary

β-Blockers	Reduce myocardial contractility
	Reduce LVH
	Advice: use if there are no signs of heart failure or other contraindication
Calcium antagonists	Reduce peripheral resistance
	Reduce LVH
	Advice: may be used safely
ACE inhibitors	Reduce peripheral resistance
	Reduce LVH
	Advice: first choice especially if there is a history of heart failure
Thiazide diuretics	Doubt about ability to reduce LVH
	Advice: may be used safely in combination with ACE inhibitors
Vasodilators	Cause reflex tachycardia
	Do not reduce LVH
	Advice: not first choice therapy

First choice: ACE inhibitors ± thiazide diuretics

Heart failure

In congestive heart failure activation of the RAA system is a frequent occurrence and increased plasma renin is commonly seen. It is important in treating hypertension with heart failure to reduce preload and afterload if possible without reducing any further the cardiac output.

Even with mild left ventricular failure, β-blockers are absolutely contra-indicated. β-Blockers reduce myocardial contractility, which reduces stroke volume and cardiac output. They also reduce heart rate, again leading to reduced cardiac output. Therefore in the presence of any existing heart failure, β-blockers serve only to worsen the situation.

Calcium antagonists such as verapamil and diltiazem should not be given because of their ability to reduce myocardial contractility and slow A-V conduction.

ACE inhibitors, on the other hand, are useful therapy, lowering blood pressure effectively while improving the overall haemodynamic picture.
ACE inhibitors decrease arterial and venous vasoconstriction, systemic vascular resistance and afterload. Aldosterone levels also decrease with a subsequent reduction in intravascular volume and preload. The net effect is a significant improvement in left ventricular performance in the majority of patients.
A modest increase in serum potassium is commonly observed but significant hyperkalaemia can be avoided by discontinuing potassium supplements and changing from potassium-sparing diuretics.

Summary

β-Blockers	Reduce myocardial contractility
	Reduce heart rate
	Advice: absolutely contraindicated
Calcium antagonists	Reduce myocardial contractility (verapamil and diltiazem in particular)
	Reduce A–V conduction
	Advice: avoid
ACE inhibitors	Reduce peripheral vascular resistance
	Reduce afterload
	Reduce intravascular volume and preload
	Advice: use as first-line therapy
Thiazide diuretics	Reduce intravascular volume
	Advice: use alone or with ACE inhibitors

First choice: ACE inhibitors + thiazide diuretic.

Ischaemic heart disease

The risk of suffering a heart attack is higher in hypertensive patients than in normotensives and it is disappointing that, so far, hypotensive treatment has failed to reduce the incidence of coronary events in hypertensive patients – the possible reasons for this were discussed earlier. Treatment must be chosen to avoid unnecessarily increasing that risk.

Diuretic drugs are used in cases of heart failure to reduce plasma volume, but care is required in using thiazide diuretics in IHD as they cause hypokalaemia in many patients, which may lead to arrhythmias.

β-blockers or calcium antagonists may be indicated to control angina, but β-blockers must not be used if there is clinical evidence of heart failure (see above). β-Blockers are a popular therapy as they can bring about a significant reduction in re-infarction rates and severity over the 2 years following a heart attack.

ACE inhibitors may be beneficial since they do not cause reflex sympathetic stimulation. They must be used with care to avoid risk of hyperkalaemia, and potassium supplements and potassium-sparing diuretics should be discontinued.

Summary

β-Blockers	Reduce myocardial contractility
	Reduce heart rate
	Advice: use if hypertension is associated with angina but not in the presence of heart failure
Calcium antagonists	Reduce myocardial contractility
	Advice: use to control angina
ACE inhibitors	Lower peripheral vascular resistance
	No reflex sympathetic stimulation
	Advice: use with care – observe serum potassium levels
Thiazide diuretics	May cause hypokalaemia
	Advice: use lowest dose available

First choice: β-blockers or ACE inhibitors according to presence of other conditions

Hyperlipidaemia

When effective antihypertensive drugs first became available it was confidently expected that their use would lead to a reduction in morbidity and mortality from ischaemic heart disease – an expectation that has not been borne out. It has now been established that some of the drugs used to treat hypertension may at the same time worsen the lipid profile of the patient, which may go some way towards explaining the disappointing impact on ischaemic heart disease seen in major trials of antihypertensive therapies.

β-Blockers are still the most commonly used antihypertensive agents, and their effects on serum lipids have been the most extensively studied. Blockade of β_2-receptors in adipose tissue reduces lipolysis, producing a fall in serum free fatty-acid concentrations. There is usually a decrease in HDL-cholesterol and an increase in triglyceride concentrations – both known to be atherogenic risk factors.

The recently introduced highly cardioselective β_1-blocker, bisoprolol, does not produce changes in glucose or lipoprotein concentrations, while labetalol, the α- and β-blocker combination, may even improve serum lipid profiles by reducing total and LDL-cholesterol and elevating HDL concentrations.

α-Blockers competitively antagonise the α-adrenoceptors which, like the β receptors, exist in two forms, α_1 and α_2. Early agents were relatively unselective and blocked α_2 sites, bringing about reflex tachycardia, fluid retention and vasoconstriction. The newer, more selective α_1 agents have fewer side-effects and also have beneficial effects on serum lipids, reducing total cholesterol, LDL-cholesterol and triglyceride levels, while increasing HDL-cholesterol.

Prazosin is unsuitable for monotherapy but terazosin and doxazosin are effective antihypertensive agents which may be used as first-line agents.

Calcium antagonists are as effective as thiazide diuretics and β-blockers at reducing blood pressure, while causing minimal metabolic side-effects. However, as yet there have been no long-term studies which show any reduction in cardiovascular morbidity or mortality using these agents.

ACE inhibitors are effective agents for controlling blood pressure, and have no adverse effects on haemodynamic functioning. Trials have not been as extensive as for some of the older agents, but those conducted so far suggest that ACE inhibitors do not significantly alter serum lipids. They may even diminish insulin resistance – a factor which has been linked to hypercholesterolaemia.

Thiazide diuretics are known to elevate plasma triglyceride levels as well as total cholesterol, although the effects are dose-related and there is some controversy over the actual risk incurred with normal therapeutic doses. Similar metabolic effects are seen, but less frequently, with loop diuretics.

Summary

β-Blockers	May elevate total cholesterol and elevate triglyceride concentrations **Advice:** avoid if possible. Use cardioselective agent for preference
α-Blockers	No adverse metabolic effects Unselective agents may cause reflex tachycardia, fluid retention and vasoconstriction Newer agents may have beneficial effects on lipid profile **Advice:** use selective agents if possible
Calcium antagonists	Minimal metabolic side-effects **Advice:** use with confidence
ACE inhibitors	No known metabolic side-effects No adverse effects on haemodynamic picture **Advice:** use with confidence
Thiazide diuretics	Elevate plasma triglyceride levels Elevate total cholesterol **Advice:** avoid unless used with ACE inhibitors

First choice: ACE inhibitors ± thiazide diuretics or α-blockers

Heart block

In heart block, the impulses from the atria to the ventricles through the A-V node are delayed or interrupted completely:

- first-degree heart block – the delayed depolarisation of the ventricles, resulting in a longer P–R interval;
- second-degree block type 1 – the conduction delay increases in subsequent beats until one impulse fails to be conducted, with the result that a beat is dropped;
- second-degree block type 2 – some depolarisation waves are conducted and some are not;
- third-degree block – atria and ventricles function completely independently of each other.

The ideal therapy for hypertension associated with heart block will reduce blood pressure by reducing peripheral resistance and will have minimal impact on cardiac function.

In most cases of heart block this effectively excludes the β-blockers, although they may be used with caution in first-degree block.

In all degrees of heart block, diuretics, calcium antagonists (excluding verapamil, which delays A–V nodal conduction) and the ACE inhibitors can be used with confidence.

Summary

β-Blockers	Reduce myocardial contractility Reduce heart rate **Advice:** avoid in second- and third-degree block
Calcium antagonists	Reduce peripheral resistance (nifedipine and nicardipine) **Advice:** use, but avoid verapamil
ACE inhibitors	Reduce peripheral resistance No effect on cardiac function **Advice:** use
Thiazide diuretics	No effect on cardiac function **Advice:** use

First choice: calcium antagonists or ACE inhibitors ± thiazide diuretics

Peripheral vascular disease

High blood pressure is often associated with peripheral vascular disease (PVD), although intermittent claudication is also common in people with normal blood pressure. Treatment may be necessary to prevent other complications but it has not been confirmed that treatment for hypertension prevents or relieves PVD.

Claudication may be induced or even worsened by treatment with β-blockers.
   β-Blockers reduce cardiac output and peripheral perfusion and also bring about increased peripheral resistance, all of which can exacerbate symptoms of pre-existing PVD.

Calcium antagonists are helpful in relieving symptoms of PVD by causing vasodilatation. Individual agents vary in their relative effects on the myocardium and on peripheral smooth muscle, nifedipine and nicardipine having a greater effect on peripheral muscle.

ACE inhibitors, with a thiazide diuretic if necessary, are a useful therapy in these patients. PVD responds well due to the ability of ACE inhibitors to bring about decreased sympathetic drive and increased compliance of large vessels. However, PVD may be a marker for renal artery stenosis and this should be excluded before ACE inhibitors are prescribed for patients with intermittent claudication or clinical signs of peripheral vascular disease – most likely in smokers and diabetics.

Summary

β-Blockers	Reduce cardiac output Reduce peripheral perfusion Increase peripheral resistance **Advice:** avoid if possible
Calcium antagonists	Reduce peripheral resistance (especially nifedipine and nicardipine) **Advice:** therapy of choice
ACE inhibitors	Reduce peripheral resistance Decrease sympathetic drive **Advice:** check for renal artery stenosis first

First choice: calcium antagonists

Asthma

β-Blockers are absolutely contraindicated in asthma as, by blocking pulmonary β_2-receptors, they may cause severe bronchial constriction. Asthmatics often use β-adrenergic agonists (e.g. salbutamol, orciprenaline, isoprenaline) to reverse bronchospasm but in the presence of β-antagonists, these β-agonists may be ineffective, and irreversible bronchospasm may occur.

α-Blockers may have some advantages in that α-blockade causes bronchodilatation. The combined α- and β-blocking drug, labetalol, has a net effect on airways resistance similar to that of the cardioselective blockers due to the bronchodilating effect of the α-blocker component.

However, in asthma, drugs with any β-blocking action should be avoided.

Calcium antagonists have no effect on bronchial smooth muscle and can be used safely by asthmatics.

ACE inhibitors are tolerated very well: they decrease hypoxic vasoconstriction and bring about an improvement in pulmonary function. They are the preferred therapy, with the addition of a thiazide diuretic if necessary.

Thiazide diuretics have no effects on airway patency and may be used safely.

Summary

β-Blockers	Block pulmonary β_2-receptors causing bronchoconstriction **Advice:** absolutely contraindicated.
α-Blockers	α-Blockade causes bronchodilatation **Advice:** use with caution
Calcium antagonists	No effect on bronchial smooth muscle **Advice:** may be used safely
ACE inhibitors	Improve pulmonary function **Advice:** therapy of choice, with diuretic if necessary
Thiazide diuretics	No effect on bronchial smooth muscle **Advice** may be used safely

First choice: ACE inhibitors $\pm$ thiazide diuretics

Diabetes mellitus

Diabetes mellitus and hypertension are common chronic disorders which frequently coexist. Hypertension appears to be almost twice as common in persons with diabetes as in those without, and diabetic clinic attenders contain an excess of hypertensives, particularly among non-insulin-dependent diabetics (type 2).

While this may be accounted for by a tendency for selective referral rather than a true association, diabetics with hypertension are a sub-group of patients particularly prone to developing serious complications. The combination is a major risk factor for early renal and cardiovascular death, and may also play a part in the emergence of diabetic complications.

There is a complex relationship between diabetes, ischaemic heart disease, hyperlipidaemia, nephropathy and peripheral disease and it is therefore particularly important to control hypertension in both types of diabetic. Treatment should be started at lower blood pressures than in other groups and requires more careful monitoring. However, treatment may not be straightforward, as hypotensive drugs can interfere with diabetic control, posing a greater risk than non-intervention.

β-Blockers. The use of β-blockers in diabetics is controversial: effects on the peripheral circulation and glucose metabolism have been well-documented, but the risks may have been over-emphasized.

β-Blockers interfere with the autonomic and metabolic response to hypoglycaemia and may therefore have disadvantages in the treatment of insulin-dependent diabetics. During hypoglycaemic episodes, hepatic glycogen stores are metabolised to glucose in an attempt to restore normal blood glucose levels. The process is under β_2-adrenergic control and β-blockers can reduce the response thus delaying recovery.

Furthermore, the symptoms of hypoglycaemia – sweating and tachycardia – are also under β_2-adrenergic control and patients using β-blockers may be unaware that they are becoming hypoglycaemic.

Blockade of pancreatic β_2-receptors brings about reduced insulin release and subsequent glucose intolerance.

Adverse effects are due predominantly to unwanted blockade of β_2 sites which theoretically should be avoided by the use of a β_1-selective agent. β_1-Specific blockers (atenolol, acebutalol and metoprolol) have fewer effects on hypoglycaemia but should be avoided in very brittle diabetics as selectivity is not total and these agents will still cause some blockade of β_2 sites.

A further consideration to bear in mind is that diabetics are particularly prone to peripheral vascular disease which may be aggravated or precipitated by β-blockers. Digital ulceration or gangrene may result.

Overall, β-blockers should be avoided in diabetics. If they must be used, they should be given in the smallest possible doses.

The α-blockers terazosin and doxazosin may improve lipid profiles while having no effect on glucose tolerance, but they are associated with a high incidence of postural hypotension and drowsiness.

Calcium antagonists have no adverse effects on lipids, potassium, glucose or uric acid levels and are safe and useful in the treatment of hypertension in diabetes.

There may be an initial slight impairment of glucose tolerance caused by impairment of glucose-stimulated insulin release, but this is not a problem with prolonged therapy.

Ankle and foot oedema are common and may lead to injury, ulceration or gangrene. The newer agents may prove to be better in this respect.

ACE inhibitors have little effect on uric acid, serum potassium, glucose or lipids, and can be administered safely to diabetic patients. However, they may enhance insulin sensitivity and the physician should be ready to reduce the dose of insulin if this happens.

Studies suggest that ACE inhibitors can reduce the hyperfiltration of protein in the glomerulus associated with diabetes, by reducing efferent arteriolar resistance.

Because of their unique mode of action ACE inhibitors appear to offer a distinct advantage in the treatment of hypertension with diabetes: they do not aggravate lipid abnormalities and also appear to protect the kidney. They are becoming favoured as first-line therapy.

Thiazide diuretics are known to be mildly diabetogenic. They inhibit insulin release from the pancreas in response to glucose challenge, and the action of insulin in enabling cellular utilization of glucose can be impeded by hypokalaemia. They are best avoided in non-insulin-dependent diabetics in case they bring about a deterioration of control.

They are not contraindicated in insulin-dependent patients although blood glucose levels will require careful monitoring at the start of therapy, and the dose of insulin may need to be increased by a small amount.
However, diabetics are at particular risk from IHD and renal failure, in contrast with non-diabetic hypertensives whose greatest risk is from stroke. Therefore, thiazide diuretics and β-blockers, which both aggravate the hyperlipidaemia often associated with diabetes, are not the first choice for reducing the risk of IHD.

Clonidine and methyldopa may be useful and have not been associated with adverse metabolic effects, but they suffer from the same adverse effects as the α-blockers, and are also associated with impotence – which may already be a problem for diabetics with neuropathy.

Summary

β-Blockers   May delay recovery from hypoglycaemia
                                     May block symptoms of hypoglycaemia
                                     May impair glucose tolerance
                                     Can adversely affect plasma lipids
                                     Can worsen peripheral ischaemia
                                     Advice: avoid

α-Blockers   No effect on glucose tolerance
                                     May cause postural hypotension and drowsiness
                                     Advice: use if tolerated

Calcium antagonists   No adverse metabolic effects
                                     May cause peripheral oedema
                                     Advice: use

ACE inhibitors   No adverse metabolic effects
                                     May enhance insulin sensitivity
                                     May reduce hyperfiltration of protein
                                     May impair renal function in cases of pre-existing renal stenosis
                                     Advice: treatment of choice

Thiazide diuretics   May impair glucose tolerance
                                     May lead to potassium depletion
                                     Can adversely affect plasma lipids
                                     Advice: avoid except with ACE inhibitors

Clonidine, methyldopa No effect on glucose tolerance
                                     May cause postural hypotension, drowsiness and impotence
                                     Advice: avoid if possible

First choice: ACE inhibitors ± thiazide diuretics

Renal failure

Once identified, cases of renal failure are unlikely to be treated in general practice: the following is for information only.

Renal disease should always be investigated to establish if there are treatable causes, but while this is happening it is important to break the vicious cycle of renal damage causing elevation of blood pressure leading to further renal damage. In patients with established chronic renal failure it is important to control blood pressure accurately, the otherwise inevitable deterioration in renal function can be delayed and some improvement may even be achieved.

β-Blockers have long been a favoured therapy as they block renin release, but they may have to be given in reduced doses, or on alternate days.

ACE inhibitors are effective in controlling hypertension in chronic renal failure, especially when used in combination with loop diuretics.

Furthermore, many studies have shown that ACE inhibitors reduce urinary protein loss in a variety of renal diseases. This may be due to a decrease in glomerular capillary pressure, leading to a reduction in filtered protein. In the long term this could retard the progression to renal function loss, but this has yet to be confirmed.

While administration of ACE inhibitors improves renal function in some patients with renal insufficiency, on rare occasions (bilateral renal artery stenosis and volume depletion associated with diuretic therapy) they may cause reversible deterioration of renal function. This is probably due to their elimination of the effect of angiotensin II on the efferent arteriole that previously maintained adequate filtration pressure. The effect is reversible on withdrawal of therapy.

If patients are dehydrated or are receiving high doses of diuretics, an over-rapid fall in blood pressure with rapid renal deterioration may occur. Diuretics should be stopped and it is best to start with the smallest possible dose, increasing it gradually.

High doses of loop diuretics may control fluid retention, particularly in combination with arterial vasodilators such as hydralazine or minoxidil. But excessive use may cause a deterioration in renal function if there is a marked reduction in blood volume and renal blood flow.

In all cases of renal failure treatment is probably best initiated in hospital.

Summary

β-Blockers	Block renin release **Advice:** use in reduced doses
ACE inhibitors	Reduce urinary protein loss May exert renoprotective effect **Advice:** the only therapy which can improve proteinuria. Use with caution in case renal failure is precipitated
Diuretics	Reduce blood volume May precipitate renal failure **Advice:** use with caution

First choice: ACE inhibitors ± thiazide diuretics

Elderly

Treatment of high blood pressure in the elderly is justified as it appears to reduce total mortality and cardiovascular disease mortality, but special efforts are required in order to avoid drug side-effects and to avoid exacerbating coexisting conditions.

The four widely-used classes of drug (thiazides, β-blockers, ACE inhibitors and calcium antagonists) have broadly similar antihypertensive efficacy so the choice of drug must be based on the presence of coexisting disease and individual tolerance.

Particular problems with the elderly are:

Postural hypotension

The elderly are likely to develop postural hypotension owing to the greater rigidity of their blood vessels and – linked with this – a decreased baroreceptor sensitivity. The likelihood of injury, and the risk of complications, is greater if such drops in blood pressure result in a fall.

Kidney

There is a decrease in the responsiveness of the renin-angiotensin system in older people, which is of little importance in itself, but could lead to a greater fall in blood pressure on a reduction in salt intake or with diuretic use. The older patient may become significantly more sodium-depleted before coming into sodium balance, providing a further risk of postural hypotension.

In the kidney, renal blood flow usually decreases with age, leading to a decrease in glomerular filtration rate. Many of the drugs used for lowering blood pressure are excreted by the kidney and may accumulate.

Catecholamines

Plasma noradrenaline levels, in contrast with plasma renin, tend to be higher in the elderly. Peripheral adrenoceptors are, however, less sensitive to catecholamines and therefore to β-blockers. These drugs are less effective in the elderly than in younger hypertensives.

Heart

Older hypertensives tend to have reduced cardiac output and lower intravascular volumes.

Heart failure is more common, probably due to a combination of ischaemic heart disease and high blood pressure. In cases of heart failure, β-blockers are contraindicated.

To summarise – the elderly hypertensive is characterized by a reduced cardiac output and renal function, with a compensatory rise in total peripheral resistance causing elevation of blood pressure.

The ideal antihypertensive agent should therefore lower arterial pressure by lowering total peripheral resistance. In addition, it should maintain systemic and target-organ blood flow and preserve cardiac performance, prevent fluid and salt retention and should not produce reflex stimulation of the sympathetic adrenergic or renin–angiotensin systems.

β-Blockers reduce cardiac output, heart rate and renal blood flow while increasing peripheral resistance. As the cardiac output of elderly patients is generally low and the peripheral resistance is high, β-blockers seem a poor choice of treatment.

In addition, the depressive and CNS effects of β-blockers may be particularly disturbing to elderly patients and there are reports that continued therapy may impair short-term memory.

Given this, β-blockers should only be prescribed to the elderly where absolutely necessary, for example, in cases of angina with hypertension. Otherwise β-blockers with intrinsic sympathomimetic activity or combined with α-blockers should be used. In this respect, labetalol may be useful, as may pindolol, with intrinsic sympathomimetic activity.

β-Blockers are well tolerated by fit elderly patients, but the higher prevalence of obstructive airways disease and peripheral vascular disease among this group reduces the number who could respond well to them.

α-Blockers (e.g. prazosin and terazosin) are best avoided as they frequently cause postural hypotension after the first dose and with subsequent increments.

Calcium antagonists are effective peripheral vasodilators, bringing about a direct decrease in total peripheral resistance. They have advantages in the treatment of the elderly in that they have no CNS side-effects, cause minimal postural hypotension, no fluid retention and maintain blood flow to crucial tissues. They do not cause bronchospasm, are not known to have significant metabolic effects, and have no significant effect on plasma insulin. They may be used in patients with coronary artery disease, diabetes or peripheral vascular disease.

Side-effects with nifedipine, such as headaches and flushing, can be controlled by starting patients on a low dose. Verapamil may cause constipation – a disadvantage for many elderly patients – and should not be used in combination with β-blockers. Peripheral oedema may cause non-compliance.

ACE inhibitors, particularly in combination with sodium restriction or a diuretic, are effective in treatment of the elderly, despite the fact that the elderly have low levels of plasma renin.

ACE inhibitors have been found to increase cerebral blood flow making them an attractive therapy for older patients.

Although the claims are still controversial, there is emerging evidence that ACE inhibitors induce a feeling of well-being in older patients and may improve the quality of life relative to other therapies.

All ACE inhibitors run the risk of bringing about first-dose hypotension, particularly if patients have also been taking diuretics but appropriate management can reduce the risk of this.

Thiazide diuretics. These have long been the cornerstone of antihypertensive treatment in the elderly, and most patients respond well to small doses. However, thiazides may cause hypokalaemia and glucose intolerance and should be used with care in patients with ischaemic heart disease, a history of myocardial infarction or receiving digoxin, as well as those known to be on a poor diet or taking laxatives. Regular monitoring is required.

Centrally-acting agents such as reserpine and methyldopa have proven efficacy in the elderly and were favoured treatments before the introduction of newer drugs. They decrease total peripheral resistance without reducing renal blood flow and with minimal changes to cardiac function, but they have largely been abandoned due to their sedative and depressive effects which may serve to aggravate confusional states.

Adrenergic neurone blockers should never be used because of the high risk of causing postural hypotension leading to falls and possible fractures.

Arterial vasodilators (e.g. hydralazine and minoxidil) produce palpitations, shortness of breath and headaches although these effects can be mitigated by the addition of a β-blocker. Arterial vasodilators do not produce orthostatic hypotension since they have no effect on the capacitance vessels. The RAA system is stimulated leading to salt and water retention, but this is more common with minoxidil, and can be overcome by addition of a loop diuretic. These are most often used in combination, as third-line agents.

Summary

β-Blockers	Reduce cardiac output
	Reduce heart rate
	Slight increase in peripheral resistance
	Reduce renal flow
	CNS effects
	Effects on peripheral vascular disease
	Advice: only use where necessary (e.g. angina with hypertension)
α-Blockers	Cause postural hypotension
	Advice: use with caution
Calcium antagonists	Reduce total peripheral resistance
	Few side-effects
	Minimal postural hypotension
	Advice: can be used with confidence (do not combine verapamil with β-blockers)
ACE inhibitors	Effective in reducing blood pressure
	May increase cerebral blood flow
	May improve 'quality of life'
	Advice: therapy of choice. Care with renal failure, and on first dose
Thiazide diuretics	Reduce blood volume
	Advice: used in small doses are effective and well-tolerated. Care with coexisting heart disease, patients taking digoxin or on poor diet
Reserpine, methyldopa	Reduce total peripheral resistance
	Minimal changes to cardiac function
	Minimal postural hypotension
	Cause sedation and depression
	Advice: avoid.
Adrenergic neurone blockers	Cause postural hypotension
	Advice: avoid
Hydralazine, minoxidil	May cause palpitations, breathlessness, headaches
	Some salt and water retention
	Advice: use only in combination

First choice: ACE inhibitors ± thiazide diuretics

Pregnancy

Bed-rest has been found to be of very little value in the control of hypertension in pregnancy. While the blood pressure may stabilise at a lower level during the resting period, as soon as the woman moves again, the pressure rises.

It is of utmost importance to try to avoid antihypertensive drugs in the first 12 weeks of pregnancy, but after this, if hypertension is severe there are a number of options.

β-Blockers and combined α-β-blockers are safe in pregnancy although there was initially some concern that β-blockers might induce bradycardia in mother and fetus. This would render the maternal and fetal heart rates less reliable when monitoring for fetal distress. However this question has now been discounted and β-blockers are the drugs of first choice in pregnant hypertensives where there are no other specific contra-indications.

The most common side-effects are cold extremities and Raynaud's phenomenon.

Calcium antagonists have been found useful in severe cases of pregnancy-associated hypertension but their use has so far been limited to controlled trials. Headaches and flushing are the major unwanted effects and about 10% of patients cannot tolerate these drugs. They tend to be used as second-line therapy.

ACE inhibitors are contraindicated in pregnancy as animal tests have been associated with decreased neonatal survival and increased likelihood of stillbirths.

Diuretics are normally contraindicated. Women with pre-eclampsia have reduced plasma volumes and diuretics will cause further contraction, which may worsen the utero-placental blood flow. Diuretics may prove necessary if there is severe heart failure or gross fluid retention due to renal failure.

Methyldopa is a centrally-acting α-receptor stimulant which causes peripheral vasodilatation by reducing sympathetic nervous system activity. It has been used for many years and is still the most widely-used drug for hypertension in pregnancy. While being safe for the fetus, there is evidence that it causes severe dose-related sedation, depression and lethargy.

94

Vasodilators have been used extensively and safely in pregnancy as second-line drugs. Side-effects include tachycardia, fluid retention and headaches.

Summary

β-Blockers	May cause cold extremities and Raynaud's phenomenon **Advice:** safe. Use with confidence
Calcium antagonists	Not well-studied Side-effects include headaches and flushing and can be intolerable **Advice:** use only in cases uncontrolled by other therapy
ACE inhibitors	**Advice:** contraindicated in pregnancy
Diuretics	May reduce plasma volume to levels which affect utero-placental blood flow **Advice:** avoid unless there is severe heart failure or gross fluid retention due to renal failure
Methyldopa	Peripheral vasodilatation Side-effects include sedation, depression, lethargy **Advice:** safe to fetus, use if tolerated
Hydralazine, minoxidil	Side-effects include tachycardia, fluid retention and headaches **Advice:** check individual product data sheets

First choice: refer to hospital

9

Combination therapy with ACE inhibitors

An ACE inhibitor used as monotherapy can be expected to control blood pressure in 30–50% of patients with essential hypertension. However, the regulatory processes which govern blood pressure control are numerous and interrelated, and the underlying cardiovascular disorder exhibits great variety. There may be differences in sympathetic drive, renin responsiveness, peripheral vascular structure, myocardial contractility, to name just a few, so it is unlikely that a single agent will be able to return a disordered cardiovascular system to normal in all patients.

It is difficult to quantify all these variables in individual patients, and it is therefore impossible to determine in advance the right drug for the right patient. As as result therapy is usually begun on an empirical basis, usually with a single agent, and other drugs are added in as appropriate.

This chapter looks at the benefits and disadvantages that can be expected when ACE inhibitors are combined with various other antihypertensive drugs.

ACE inhibitor + diuretic

Hypotensive activity

Diuretics achieve hypotension by eliminating salt and water, thus reducing blood volume. The renin–angiotensin system is immediately stimulated as a reflex response in order to conserve blood volume.

When ACE inhibitors are used at the same time, activation of the renin–angiotensin system is prevented, enhancing the effect of both therapies. An impressive synergistic effect often results when low-dose ACE inhibitors are combined in this way with thiazide diuretics.

Side-effects

The metabolic side-effects of diuretic therapy such as hyperuricaemia, hyper-cholesterolaemia and hyperglycaemia are all attenuated during combination therapy with ACE inhibitors, while plasma potassium levels are usually maintained due to the reduction of aldosterone secretion. Potassium-sparing diuretics are therefore not usually required and indeed may even precipitate hyperkalaemia.

On the other hand, loop diuretics have been used effectively in combination therapy without causing disturbances in electrolyte levels.

Black patients tend to have lower renin levels than white and show a lesser response to ACE inhibitor therapy, but this difference is abolished by the concomitant use of a diuretic.

Overall, hypertension may be controlled in 80% of patients with a combination of ACE inhibitor and thiazide diuretic.

ACE inhibitor + calcium antagonist

Calcium antagonists may induce tachycardia in a reflex increase of symp-athetic activity while ACE inhibitors, by increasing vagal activity, can counteract this effect.

Calcium antagonists have a consistent synergistic effect when used in combination with ACE inhibitors. Both drugs improve compliance of the large arteries, an especially desirable feature in the elderly.

Reports have shown nifedipine to be an effective combination with ACE inhibitors in very resistant hypertension.

ACE inhibitor + β-blocker

β-Blockers inhibit renin release, and ACE inhibitors block the formation of angiotensin II. Overall, the effects of both drugs on this system are very similar and there is little to gain from using them in combination. Trials suggest that the combination could, in fact, be less than additive.

10

Conclusion

ACE inhibitors are now firmly established for use in general practice but there is still some uncertainty amongst doctors about their precise role and application. This is entirely understandable and reflects the healthy conservatism of general practitioners faced with new drugs.

The unease about the ACE inhibitors was exacerbated in the early days by problems with the recommended dosage which was initially set too high, and frequently caused severe side-effects. This has now been resolved, severe side-effects are rare and the drugs are well tolerated by the majority of patients.

Hypertension and heart failure, for which ACE inhibitors are now in regular use, are both long-term chronic conditions treated in general practice. It is therefore of particular importance that GPs feel confident in their use.

ACE inhibitors are already the first choice of drug for hypertension in certain groups of patients. They are particularly useful in diabetics, the elderly and where β-blockers are contraindicated. The list may increase in the future when the results of further studies are available.

In heart failure it is now usual to start an ACE inhibitor as soon as the smallest dose of diuretic becomes inadequate in controlling symptoms. This means that, within a short time, a very large number of patients, particularly the elderly, will be taking a combination of ACE inhibitor and diuretic.

Accurate initial diagnosis both of the heart failure and its underlying cause are of paramount importance. Hospital referral may be necessary to sort this out.

At present, there is little to choose between the different preparations available, although further research may in the future show significant differences in efficacy. Since treatment is often initiated in hospital, the choice of drug is usually in the hands of the hospital consultants.

The most important aspect of the long-term management of patients with chronic heart failure is monitoring treatment. This can be carried out effectively only in general practice, where drug treatment can be titrated against levels of activity, quality of life and biochemical parameters. Clear protocols for this are needed at practice level for the use of the members of the primary health-care team.

Similarly, the long-term management of hypertension needs monitoring which can effectively only be done in general practice.

These aspects of patient care are now well within the capabilities of general practitioners but long-term monitoring is complex and requires careful organisation. We hope that this book has helped to clarify the place of the ACE inhibitor drugs in modern therapy.

Further Reading

Beevers DG, MacGregor GA. Hypertension in practice. Martin Dunitz Ltd; 1987.

Messerli FH, Swales JD, eds. Hypertension and the elderly. Science Press Ltd; 1989.

Strube G, Strube G. Commonsense Cardiology. Kluwer Academic Publishers, Lancaster; 1989.

Index

ACTH (corticotrophin) 57
adrenaline 4
adrenergic neurone blockers 92, 93
agranulocytosis 72
alcohol consumption 19
aldosterone 10, 11, 57
    ACE inhibitor actions 60
α adrenergic effects 4, 5
α-blockers
    asthma 84
    diabetes 86, 87
    elderly 91, 93
    hyperlipidaemia 80, 81
aminopeptidase 57
angina 28, 79
angioneurotic oedema 71
angiotensin converting enzyme
    (ACE) 9, 11, 55, 57, 59
    tissue 63
angiotensin converting enzyme
    (ACE) inhibitors 1–2, 10,
    52, 55–67, 99–100
    asthma 84
    clinical effects 61–5
    combination therapy 97–8
    contraindications 73
    diabetes 86, 87
    dosage 67
    early problems 56, 69
    elderly 72, 92, 93
    first-dose response 71
    heart block 82
    heart failure 63, 66–7, 73, 78,
    99–100
    history of development 55–6
    hyperlipidaemia 80, 81
    indications 66–7
    ischaemic heart disease 79
    left ventricular hypertrophy 63,
    76, 77
    mode of action 59–61
    peripheral vascular disease 83
    pharmacodynamics 66
    pharmacokinetics 65
    precautions 72–3
    pregnancy 94, 95
    renal disease 72, 73, 88, 89
    safety 69–73
    side-effects 70–2
    vs. other antihypertensives
    69–70
angiotensin I 9, 56–7
angiotensin II 9–10, 17, 57
    action of ACE inhibitors 60
    actions 10, 62
angiotensinogen 9, 56
antidiuretic hormone (ADH) 10,
    11, 57, 61
antihypertensive drugs
    ACE inhibitors *vs.* 69–70
    combination therapy 97–8
    sites of action 13, 14
    special patient groups 75–95
    see also specific types of drugs

aorta
    coarctation 39
    effects of hypertension 22
arteries
    ACE inhibitor therapy and 63
    effects of hypertension 17-18,
        21-2
asthma, antihypertensive therapy
    84
atheroma 20
atheromatous plaques 23
autonomic nervous system 4-6, 7,
    62

bendrofluazide 51
β adrenergic effects 4, 5
β-blockers 1, 6, 51
    and ACE inhibitors combined
        98
    ACE inhibitors vs. 69-70
    asthma 84
    diabetes 85, 87
    elderly 91, 93
    heart block 82
    heart failure 78
    hyperlipidaemia 80, 81
    ischaemic heart disease 79
    left ventricular hypertrophy 76,
        77
    peripheral vascular disease 83
    pregnancy 94, 95
    renal failure 88, 89
bisoprolol 80
blood dyscrasias 72
blood pressure
    ACE inhibitors and 61
    control in emergency states
        12-13
    diastolic, normal distribution
        24, 26
    life expectancy and 24, 25
    measurement 36
    physiological control 3-13
    records 34, 35

systolic, degree of risk and 24,
    26
bone marrow depression 72
bradykinin 11, 61
brain, effects of hypertension 22

calcium antagonists 1, 51-2
    and ACE inhibitors combined
        98
    ACE inhibitors vs. 70
    asthma 84
    diabetes 86, 87
    elderly 91-2, 93
    heart block 82
    heart failure 78
    hyperlipidaemia 80, 81
    ischaemic heart disease 79
    left ventricular hypertrophy 76,
        77
    peripheral vascular disease 83
    pregnancy 94, 95
captopril 56, 65, 66, 67
catecholamines 4, 10, 90
cerebral haemorrhage 22
cerebral infarction 22
cerebrovascular accident, see stroke
cholesterol 13-15, 45
    total (TC) 13, 15
claudication, intermittent,
        antihypertensive therapy 83
clonidine 86, 87
coarctation of aorta 39
combination drug therapy 97-8
computer systems, hypertension
        screening 33
Conn's syndrome 39
coronary artery disease, see
        ischaemic heart disease
corticotrophin (ACTH) 57
cough 70-1
Cushing's syndrome 39

dementia 22
diabetes mellitus
   antihypertensive therapy 85–7
   hypertension 20–1
diet, healthy 45–7
diuretics
   and ACE inhibitors combined
      72, 97–8
   loop 88, 98
   pregnancy 94, 95
   renal failure 88, 89
   thiazide, see thiazide diuretics

ECG measurement 41
elderly
   ACE inhibitor therapy 72, 92,
      93
   antihypertensive therapy 90–3
   blood pressure measurement 36
   need for treatment of
      hypertension 28–9
enalapril 56, 65, 66, 67
examination, patient 40
exercise 3, 45
exertion, intense 12

family history, hypertension 20
fats, blood 13–15, 45, 80
Friedwald formula 15
ganglion-blocking agents 1
glomerular filtration rate (GFR) 9,
   73

haemorrhage 12
health education 43–7
health promotion clinics 33
heart
   effects of ACE inhibitors 61, 63
   effects of hypertension 21
   elderly 91
heart block, antihypertensive
      therapy 82

heart failure 24, 28
   ACE inhibitor therapy 63, 66–7,
      73, 78, 99–100
   antihypertensive therapy 78
   elderly 91
height–weight chart 46
hepatic disease, ACE inhibitor
      therapy 73
high-density lipoprotein (HDL) 13,
   15
history taking 39
hydralazine 92, 93, 95
hyperkalaemia 72
hyperlipidaemia, antihypertensive
      therapy 80–1
hypersensitivity reactions 71
hypertension
   assessment 37–41
   causative factors 18–21
   diagnostic criteria 36–7
   drug treatment 49–52
      ACE inhibitors 66
      drug plan 51–2
      mild hypertension 49
      moderate and severe
         hypertension 50–1
      special patient groups 75–95
      see also antihypertensive
         drugs
   effects on target organs 21–4
   essential 31–41
   long-term monitoring 52–4, 100
   need for treatment 24–9
   non-drug treatment 48–9
   old age 28–9
   pathophysiology 17–18
   prevalence 26–8
   screening 33–4, 38
   secondary 39
   setting for management 31, 32
   systolic 28
   treatment 47–52
hypertensive encephalopathy 22

hypotension
    first-dose ACE
        inhibitor-induced 71
    postural 90

indapamide 76
index card system, hypertension
    screening 33
investigations 40–1
ischaemic heart disease 22
    antihypertensive therapy 79
    benefits of treatment of
        hypertension 24, 28, 80
    risk factors 18–19

kallikrein–kinin system 11, 61
kidneys
    ACE inhibitor therapy and
        61–2
    angiotensin II actions 57
    elderly 90
    hypertension and 24
kininase II 11, 55

labetalol 80, 84
left ventricular hypertrophy (LVH)
    21
    ACE inhibitor therapy 63, 76,
        77
    antihypertensive therapy 76–7
    ECG signs 41
left ventricular output (LVO) 3
life expectancy, blood pressure and
    24, 25
lipids, blood 13–15, 45, 80
lipoproteins 13–15
lisinopril 65, 66, 67
loop diuretics 88, 98
low-density lipoprotein (LDL) 13,
    15, 45

medical records 34, 35
methyldopa 1
    diabetes 86, 87

elderly 92, 93
    pregnancy 94, 95
minoxidil 92, 93, 95
myocardial infarction 2, 21, 28

nifedipine 51–2
non-steroidal anti-inflammatory
    drugs (NSAIDs) 70–1
noradrenaline 4, 90
nurses, practice 52, 53, 54

obesity 45
optic fundus examination 40

parasympathetic nervous system
    6, 7
perindopril 65, 66, 67
peripheral resistance 3
peripheral vascular disease,
        antihypertensive therapy 83
phaeochromocytoma 39
pregnancy, antihypertensive therapy
    94–5
prostaglandins 11, 61

quinapril 65, 66, 67

ramipril 65, 66, 67
recall system 52
renal artery stenosis 10, 62, 73
renal disease
    ACE inhibitor therapy 72, 73,
        88, 89
    antihypertensive therapy 88–9
    hypertension and 24, 39
renin 9, 10, 56, 59
    plasma activity (PRA) 60
    serum levels in hypertension 19
renin–angiotensin–aldosterone
        system (RAAS)
    control of blood pressure 9–11
    function 59
    haemorrhage 12
    local endogenous 9, 63–4

renin–angiotensin–aldosterone
    system *(continued)*
  pathophysiology of hypertension
    17–18
  physiology 56–9
reserpine 92, 93

salt intake 19, 49
screening, hypertension 33–4, 38
smoking 20
  health education 44
  passive 44
special patient groups 75–95
stress 20
stroke (cerebrovascular accident)
    2, 21, 22, 24, 28
subarachnoid haemorrhage 22
sympathetic nervous system 4–6, 57
  emergency states 12
  α and β effects 4, 5
  pathophysiology of hypertension
    17–18
systemic vascular resistance
    (SVR) 3

taste 71
thiazide diuretics 1
  ACE inhibitors *vs.* 70
  asthma 84
  diabetes 86, 87
  elderly 92, 93
  heart block 82
  heart failure 78
  hyperlipidaemia 81
  ischaemic heart disease 79
  left ventricular hypertrophy 76,
    77
triglycerides 15, 45

vagal tone 6
vasodilators 76, 77, 92, 95
vasopressin (antidiuretic hormone,
    ADH) 10, 11, 57, 61
very-low-density lipoprotein
    (VLDL) 15

weight control 45, 46